Omega-3 Handbook

A ready reference guide for health professionals

Omega-3 Handbook

A Ready Reference Guide for Health Professionals

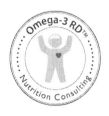

Gretchen K. Vannice, MS, RD

Disclaimer
This publication contains the opinions and ideas of its author. The information contained in this book is intended to provide helpful and informative material on the subject addressed. It is not intended to serve as a replacement for professional medical advice. The author specifically disclaims all responsibility for any liability, loss, or risk, personal or otherwise, which is incurred through the use and applications of any of the contents of this book.

ISBN-13:
978-1-46-633913-2

ISBN-10:
1-46-633913-6

Jill Kelly, PhD, editor
JiEun Park, graphic designer
Masha Shubin, interior layout
Chris Moore, web designer

Portland, Oregon

4 5 6 7 8 9 10 11 12

Dedicated to those who understand the fundamental role of nutrition in disease prevention and healthcare and the powerful influence it has on the quality of our lives.

Acknowledgements

Omega-3 Handbook would not have been completed without the help and support of Jill Kelly, PhD, the best editor a person could ask for; Leslie Kay, MS, RD colleague and friend; and my sister Michelle VanNice.

Additional thanks to:
- These senior scientists in fatty acid nutrition: Susan Carlson, Philip Calder, Bill and Sonja Connor, Claudio Galli, Bill Harris, Captain Joe Hibbeln, Penny Kris-Etherton, Norman Salem, and Charlie Serhan, for their pioneering efforts in the field and for being my teachers and mentors, beyond the textbook.
- These colleagues and their valuable feedback: Dorothy Humm, MS, RD, Marisa Castaldini, MS, RD and Jan Adams, MS, RD.
- Kelley Fitzpatrick, MS, for her contributions and expertise on plant-based omega-3s, and JiEun Park, graphic designer.

And a special thanks to the fish and marine life that bring us these unique nutrients.

Table Contents

A Note to My Colleagues

The idea for this ready reference handbook began after I gave presentations and fielded questions from dietitians and other health professionals. Between the research findings, the products available, and the claims flooding the marketplace, I saw the confusion and I understood it. Then a new drug made from fish oil was approved. I work with omega-3s every day and it was hard to stay abreast of all the information.

For 10 years, I've been working with omega-3 fatty acids in academia, industry, and healthcare. I've educated physicians, seen the inside of the fish oil industry, heard lectures from leading experts, and I'm a consumer, too. Omega-3s are not simple. They just aren't. *Form* and *source* and *dose* matter.

What I know is this: We cannot be passive about omega-3s in nutrition and health; the impact they have is worth the effort to ensure sufficient intake for our clients, friends, and families.

Improving intake of long-chain omega-3s will reduce the burden of disease and the cost of healthcare.

To quote my statistics professor, "Make things as simple as possible and not any simpler." That's what I've attempted to do with the *Omega-3 Handbook*.

I look forward to hearing from you.

Gretchen Vannice, MS, RD
Portland, Oregon
September 2011

Where the Story Begins

The omega-3 story began in the late 1960s when a Danish doctor and his student made a research journey to Greenland. At that time, death from heart disease among men aged 45 to 64 was over 40% in the United States and about 35% in Denmark, but only 5.3% in Greenland.

Confounding this mystery was knowledge that the Greenland Eskimos consumed a high fat diet, comprised largely of seal and whale blubber.

Dr. H.O. Bang and his student, Jorn Dyerberg, traveled to Illorsuit Island, Greenland, on a quest to uncover this mystery. They were warmly welcomed by the villagers; one community consisted of about 200 people and 900 sled dogs. Dr. Dyerberg, now in his 80s, speaks of these travels as a grand adventure. Very exciting for a young doctor! They were able to collect blood samples and process them in a temporary on-site laboratory. When they returned to Denmark, they compared the samples with Danish controls. The findings were surprising.

Both groups consumed about the same amount of fat in their diets, nearly 40%. The Eskimos consumed more cholesterol. In their blood, the Eskimos had higher levels of saturated fat but lower levels of polyunsaturated fat, cholesterol and triglycerides. They also had nearly 3 times the amount of omega-3s and 1/3 the amount of omega-6s. In particular, the doctors noted high levels of a relatively unknown fatty acid called EPA (up to 16% in plasma).

Thus, the prevailing notion that a high fat diet would increase risk for heart disease could not be explained here.

When the study authors published this work in the 1970s, they concluded, "It is suggested instead to be a special metabolic effect of the long chain polyunsaturated fatty acids from marine mammals."

For more information, see Resources

If dietary differences are the main reasons for the differences in ischemic heart disease incidence in Eskimos, the results from the present study point more toward qualitative than toward quantitative differences in respect of fatty acid composition of the food.

J. Dyerberg et al., 1975

CHAPTER 1

An Introduction to Omega-3s

Omega-3s are one of the most studied nutrients around the globe. There are multiple forms of these essential components of health, and multiple sources. They are essential in basic nutrition and can be used therapeutically. They were first available in foods, then in supplements, and now through a variety of fortified foods; there are prescription drugs made from fish oil and more are being developed.

Omega-3s are not vitamins or minerals; instead, they are essential fatty acids. They are required in human nutrition and the body cannot make them but must consume them, hence the term *essential*. Humans must rely on food sources or supplementation to meet this nutritional need.

Nearly all Americans get plenty of fat in their diet, many even get plenty of polyunsaturated fats, but most do not get enough omega-3. Here's why: Processed foods are primarily manufactured with vegetable oil that supplies omega-6 fatty acids, so from those foods plus meat and dairy products, most of us get an abundance of omega-6 fats in the diet. Those eating healthier food plans with plenty of olive oil are getting the monounsaturated fat, omega-9. But the body also needs a steady and sufficient intake of omega-3 fatty acids to support good health. Whether it is recommending omega-3 fatty acids for basic nutrition, for disease prevention, or therapeutic use, understanding the differences in form, source, and dose will help you guide your clients with clarity. Distinguishing the differences in form, source, and dose is central for achieving their health goals.

Table 1-1 Health Evidence-at-a-Glance: Long-Chain Omega-3s

Strongest evidence	*Emerging* evidence
• Cardiovascular disease	• Cognitive health
• Infant development	• Diabetes type 2
• Maternal health	• Weight management
• Mental health	• Immune diseases
• Rheumatoid arthritis	• Renal conditions
• Child & adolescent health	• Athletic recovery
• Vision	
• Hypertension	
• Metabolic syndrome	

RESEARCH OVERVIEW

Thousands of clinical research trials have documented the extensive health benefits of EPA and DHA, the two most functionally important omega-3 essential fatty acids. Simply stated, EPA and DHA are involved in the cellular mechanics of every cell in the human body. These long-chain omega-3s are central to healthy nutrition and preventing heart disease. They play vital roles in heart and circulatory health. They are implicated in maintaining normal blood pressure, managing inflammation, and supporting cognitive health as we age. And recently, they have been associated with improving biological age and longevity[1].

They're important nutrients for other reasons as well. Many experts consider DHA an essential nutrient in infant development and maternal health. There is keen interest in the role of EPA and DHA for psychiatric conditions. Evidence suggests they are important in immune health and endocrine function though the science is still emerging. And since long-chain omega-3s specifically provide structural as well as metabolic functions in the human brain and eye, consuming them supports the health of these organs at all stages of life, including during pregnancy.

THE FOUR OMEGA-3S

There are four commonly occurring omega-3 fatty acids: EPA, DHA, ALA, and SDA. EPA and DHA are most easily obtained from fish and marine sources, such as cold-water fish and seafood. (See Chapter 2 for values of EPA and DHA in commonly consumed fish.) ALA naturally occurs in plants (e.g., flax seed, walnuts, soybeans) while SDA naturally occurs in a little known plant-sourced echium oil although SDA has been genetically modified into the soybean and will soon be available on the market. ALA, SDA, EPA, and DHA are chemically similar (thus all are named omega-3 fats), yet they differ in their contribution to human metabolism and physiology. Table 1-2 lists nomenclature information about these long-chain fatty acids.

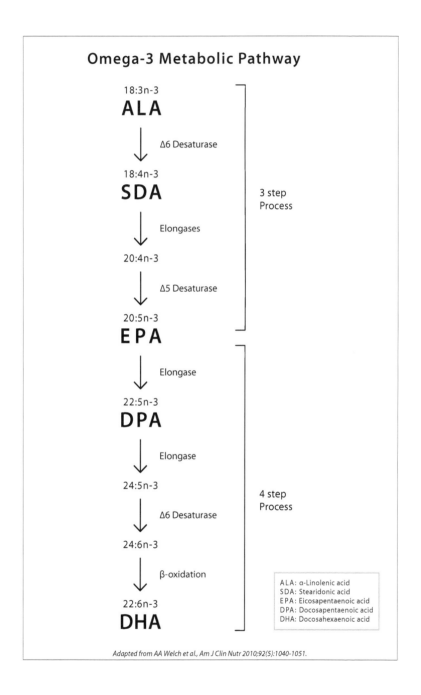

Omega-3 Metabolic Pathway

Adapted from AA Welch et al., Am J Clin Nutr 2010;92(5):1040-1051.

Table 1-2 Nomenclature of Select Fatty Acids

Name	Nomenclature
Long-chain	
DHA (docosahexaenoic acid)	22:6n-3
EPA (eicosapentaenoic acid)	20:5n-3
Short-chain	
SDA (stearidonic acid)	18:4n-3
ALA (alpha linolenic acid)	18:3n-3
Long-chain	
ARA (arachidonic acid)	20:4n-6
Short-chain	
GLA (gamma linolenic acid)	18:3n-6
LA (linoleic acid)	18:2n-6

ALA/SDA AND CONVERSION

ALA has long been considered *the* dietary essential omega-3 fatty acid in the US, based on the fact that ALA can be converted to EPA and DHA. In nutrition and chemistry textbooks, the metabolic pathway diagrams begin with ALA as the parent omega-3. (See Omega-3 Metabolic Pathway figure on opposite page.) However, substantial animal and human research in the past decade has demonstrated that ALA is not a reliable source of DHA, and to a lesser extent, of EPA for humans because the conversion rate from ALA to EPA and DHA in the body is poor[2,3].

Here's what we're learning: In order for the shorter-chain omega-3s, such as ALA and SDA, to function in the body as EPA or DHA, they must undergo metabolic

Table 1-3 Forms of Omega-3 and Their Sources

Form of omega-3	Plant foods	Marine foods	Fortified foods	Dietary supplements
ALA	Yes		Yes	Yes
SDA	Yes		Yes	
EPA		Yes	Yes	Yes
DPA		Yes		
DHA		Yes	Yes	Yes

conversion. Conversion involves elongation (adding carbons) and desaturation (adding double bonds). And, unfortunately, in humans, this conversion is inefficient. The rate of conversion of ALA to EPA is about 5% (an average range of 5–15%) and the rate of conversion of ALA to DHA is even lower (~0.5%)[1] (an average range of 0.1–3%). Women do convert ALA to DHA somewhat more efficiently than men, and women tend to have slightly higher levels of DHA than men, but the difference isn't significant.

Stearidonic acid (SDA) has 18 carbons like ALA but it has 4 double bonds while ALA has 3. SDA is thus one step closer to becoming EPA, eliminating the need for the first conversion step. The rates of conversion of SDA to EPA have been measured to be about 17%, but rate of conversion of SDA to DHA of zero[4,5].

In sum, while plant source omega-3s can supply modest yet valuable amounts of EPA, they are unable to supply efficacious tissue levels of DHA in humans[1,2]. Conversion is further impaired by genetic influences, health conditions, dietary intake of other fatty acids, etc.

BIOLOGICAL FUNCTIONS OF EPA
AND DHA: A BRIEF OVERVIEW

EPA functions in cell membranes as an eicosanoid; it is a precursor to prostaglandins, leukotrienes, and thromboxanes. Eicosanoids are regulatory molecules, functioning to maintain homeostasis in hundreds of metabolic pathways, including inflammation, vasoconstriction, platelet aggregation, and more. Arachidonic acid (ARA), an often-mentioned omega-6 found in meat and animal foods, is also an eicosanoid. Much of EPA's importance in human nutrition lies in maintaining a healthy cellular balance with ARA. Together and competitively, EPA and ARA regulate many physiologically important cellular functions[6,7].

DHA makes unique contributions to human growth and development both in terms of structure and regulation of activities. Distinctive for its chemical structure (e.g., fatty acid chain length, number of double bonds), DHA is the preferred fatty acid in eyes, brain cells, and sperm. Specifically concentrated in membrane lipids (fat) of the brain's gray matter and in the visual elements of the eye's retina, DHA is the most abundant omega-3 fatty acid in the central nervous system[8]. For reference, 14% of total fatty acids in brain cell membranes are DHA and 19% of total fatty acids as DHA has been reported in the retina of humans[9,10]. Brain composition of DHA is dependent on diet, and this begins during fetal development[11,12].

Finally, a new role for EPA and DHA as active mediators in the resolution of inflammation is emerging, and as such they are called *resolvins* and *protectins*[13].

INTAKE AND RECOMMENDATIONS

When the US Institute of Medicine established Dietary

Reference Intakes for total fat and fatty acids in 2002, they set an Adequate Intake for ALA omega-3 for men and women at 1.6 and 1.1 grams per day, respectively, with approximately 10% as EPA and DHA[14]. The Adequate Intake was set based on the "highest median intake for ALA by adults in the US where a deficiency is basically non-existent in noninstitutionalized populations"[14]. Estimated intakes of ALA, EPA. and DHA in the US adult population can be seen in Table 1-4. On average, Americans are consuming 90–110 mg EPA and DHA omega-3 per day. (See Resources for recommendations on intake from a variety of health organizations.) In short, all of the national health organizations that have set recommendations recommend that adults eat fish two or more times a week. Children should follow guidelines for adults.

A minimum intake of 250-500 mg EPA and DHA is recommended for everyone.

Table 1-4 Estimated Mean Intakes of Omega-3 Fatty Acids, United States[*][15]

Omega-3 fatty acid	Mg/day
ALA	1300 - 1330
EPA	28 - 40
DHA	57 - 70

---

*   Source: NHANES III and CSFII[15]

General Guidelines for Recommending Intake of Omega-3

Step 1. <u>Assess the diet</u>.
Most people fall into 3 categories:
1. Those who eat fish regularly (likely meet baseline nutrition needs)
2. Those who eat fish infrequently (may need to include supplement or fortified foods)
3. Those who don't or won't eat fish (consider supplement or fortified foods)

Step 2. <u>Complete a nutrition assessment.</u>
There are many factors to consider.
Is your client:
- At risk for under-consumption?
- At risk for heart disease?
- At risk for metabolic syndrome?
- Pregnant or planning to get pregnant?
- Responsible for feeding children?
- Responsible for family meal planning?

Consider testing for omega-3 blood levels

Step 3. <u>Make recommendations.</u>
1. Review recommendations by national health organizations (see Resources)
2. Complete the client assessment.
   a. Factors to consider include age, dietary intake, personal preferences, lifestyle habits, health history, and your nutrition assessment.
   b. Consider if your clients' heath needs are for:
      I. Baseline nutrition (Follow recommendations by ADA)

       II. Prevention (Follow recommendations by AHA, APA)

       III. Therapeutic intervention (Consult with physician)

  3. Present and discuss best recommendations.

     a. Recommendations should be specific by *form* and *dose* and *duration* (Note: It is a healthy practice to include plant forms of omega-3 as part of a balanced diet.

  4. Plan follow-up consult, include retesting as appropriate

ADA = American Dietetic Association
AHA = American Heart Association
APA = American Psychiatric Association

INCREASING BLOOD LEVELS OF EPA AND DHA

Ingesting EPA and DHA omega-3 raises blood and tissue levels, and that has been well documented. Increases in plasma levels can be seen within hours of consumption, but to see meaningful changes in red blood cell membranes, it takes 3-4 months. This is also true in regard to changes in brain levels. This explains why it takes regular consumption of sufficient amounts of long-chain omega-3 over time to experience benefits in mental health or arthritic conditions, for example. These are fat-soluble nutrients and it takes time for tissue levels to change. The good news is that with compliance and sufficient dose, tissue levels will increase. The alternative is true, as well. When consumption of EPA and DHA from diet or supplements is stopped, tissue levels fall.

Table 1-5 Estimated** Dose and Time to Increase Blood Levels[16]

Dose of EPA + DHA	Time
1 g/day	24 week
2 g/day	12 weeks
3 g/day	8 weeks

MEASURING OMEGA-3 BLOOD LEVELS

Measuring one's omega-3 levels requires a blood test. In recent years, tests have become available that measure omega-3 fatty acid levels. These tests use a finger-prick method, are validated, and provide a full fatty acid profile. Two companies that provide the tests are the HS-Omega-3

---

*   Estimated requirements to increase red blood cell membrane levels by 4%.

Index® (www.Omegaquant.com) and Holman Omega-3 Test® (www.omega3test.com).

Table 1-6 Actual Change in RBC Membrane Levels of EPA and DHA after Supplementation[†][17]

Patient	Baseline level[*]	Level at 12 weeks	Increase
54y male, vegetarian diet	3.80%	6.30%	2.50%
37y female, regular diet	4.50%	7.30%	2.80%
18y male, junk food diet	5.10%	7.90%	2.80%

Abbreviation: y = age in years

[†] Supplementation with 2.2 g EPA and DHA in concentrated fish oil capsules

[*] Percent of EPA and DHA in RBC membranes measured by HS-Omega-3 Index®

THE IMPORTANCE OF A HEALTHY RATIO OF OMEGA-3 TO OMEGA-6

Both omega-3 and omega-6 fatty acids are dietary essential fatty acids. And in earlier times, diets, especially along the coasts, included a more balanced supply of both. Today, due to advances in food manufacturing, North Americans consume much larger quantities of omega-6 fats and much lower quantities of omega-3 compared to 100 years ago. At the same time, over these 100 years, we've had significant increases in chronic disease, obesity, and other inflammatory-related health conditions.

Omega-6s tend to be pro-inflammatory in the body and omega-3s anti-inflammatory; they work in tandem and when the balance is good, the body functions better.

Our cells thus reflect our diet. Since our bodies cannot make omega-3 and omega-6 fats, we must get them from the food we eat. There is a current abundance of omega-6 in the North American diet from packaged foods, vegetable oils, meat,

> EPA and DHA tissue levels are independent risk factors for important cardiovascular outcomes, such as sudden cardiac death and total mortality*.
>
> ───────────────
>
> * Harris WS. The Omega-3 Index: Clinical Utility for Therapeutic Intervention. Curr Cardiol Rep. 2010;12:503–508.

chicken, and dairy foods. The predominant omega-6 fat in our diet, about 90%, is linoleic acid. An estimated 7–10% of all calories in the US food supply come from linoleic acid (note that is % of total calories, not % of fat calories)[18,19,20].

Here are some points to consider:

- More omega-6 in the diet interferes with conversion of shorter-chain omega-3s (ALA and SDA) to longer-chain omega-3s (EPA and DHA) due to enzyme competition. This is particularly relevant for vegans and vegetarians.
- More omega-6 in the diet displaces tissue levels of omega-3.
- More omega-6 in the diet does not simply mean more inflammation. Some omega-6 fats can be anti-inflammatory.
- Omega-6s are important to the healthy diet. The issue is one of increasing omega-3 fats and not consuming an overabundance of any kind of fat, which can lead to obesity.
- Keep in mind that our ancestors didn't consume

large quantities of refined oil from corn, sunflower, and soybeans; they were eating these nutritious grains, seeds, and beans as whole foods.

The best action we can take is to Keep It Simple and advise our clients to do the following:
1. Increase overall intake of omega-3s in the diet.
2. Aim for at least 500 mg EPA and DHA per day or more.
3. Limit consumption of refined, processed foods.

SAFETY CONSIDERATION: BLOOD THINNING

The concerns over increased risk of blood thinning are based largely on our understanding of mechanisms of action with long-chain omega-3 and omega-6 fatty acids. In normal, healthy individuals, supplementing up to 3000 mg EPA and DHA per day from fish oil is considered safe with no significant risk of increased bleeding time[21]. However, doses greater than 3 grams per day can inhibit blood coagulation and potentially increase the risk of bleeding[22]. Individuals on anticoagulation therapy should be monitored periodically.

A review of 19 studies with cardiac patients given between 1–4 grams of EPA and DHA from fish oil reported the risk for clinically significant bleeding was "virtually nonexistent"[23]. The Natural Medicines Comprehensive Database gives fish oil and anticoagulant/antiplatelet drugs an interaction rating of *Minor* based on a B level of evidence[22].

In North America, it is common for patients to be advised to stop fish oil supplementation 2 weeks prior to surgery.

> Dose-response between marine-source EPA and DHA omega-3s and triglyceride lowering: an approximate 5-10% reduction in triglycerides for every 1 gram of EPA and DHA consumed*.
>
> ───────────
>
> * Miller M, et al. Triglycerides and cardiovascular disease: A scientific statement from the American Heart Association. *Circulation* 2011;123:2292-2333.

FREQUENTLY ASKED QUESTIONS

Why are they called omega-3s?

The name has to do with the location of the first double bond in the polyunsaturated fatty acid chain. In omega-3s, the first double bond occurs at the third carbon molecule from the omega end; in omega-6 fats, that first double bond is at the sixth carbon molecule from the omega end.

Does fish oil have GRAS status?

Yes, the FDA has established a GRAS (Generally Regarded as Safe) level at 3 grams of EPA and DHA per day[9]. Note that is 3 grams of EPA and DHA, not 3 grams of fish or marine oil.

Do I recommend more EPA or DHA?

For general nutrition, it is best to recommend good amounts of both EPA and DHA in the diet, from food or supplements. Consuming a significant amount of more EPA than DHA or vice versa may become relevant when using omega-3s therapeutically, though the science delineating the differ-ence is still young. There is preliminary evidence suggesting that, for example, in conditions such as depression and arthritis, consuming relatively more EPA is helpful, though having sufficient DHA is also important. Conversely, DHA has been associated with cognition as we age[24,25,26,27,28].

Can we get too much EPA and DHA?

We don't know. On average, North Americans have about 4 % EPA and DHA in their red blood cell membranes, and this level is associated with a relatively high risk for sudden car-diac death. The Japanese, who are regular fish consumers, have an average EPA and DHA level of 9.5%. In the 1960s, Greenland Eskimos had 11% EPA and DHA in their plasma phospholipids. In my working knowledge, the highest level was a nutrition scientist whose blood levels were 18% with no observable adverse effects[29]. A level considered too high hasn't been clearly identified, perhaps because the bigger problem most of us face are blood levels that are too low. There is likely a level at which displacement of other fatty acids could be problematic.

The FDA has established a GRAS (Generally Regarded as Safe) level at 3 grams of EPA and DHA per day[9]. Measuring blood level is the best way to learn one's omega-3 levels. EPA and DHA red blood cell levels of 8% or higher are considered protective from death from coronary heart disease[30,31,32,33.].

Can we get too much of either EPA or DHA?

Again, we don't know. EPA converts to DHA through a complex and rare metabolic process (2 elongase steps in a row). DHA can retro-convert to EPA, though not very efficiently (about 10%), so there is an inherent check-and-balance system in place in the body.

How long do I wait to test changes in blood levels after dietary changes?

It takes about 4 months to see meaningful changes in red blood cell membranes. It's best to allow at least 4-6 months between tests.

I have heard omega-3s described as hormones. Are they?

As noted above, EPA omega-3 and ARA omega-6 are eicosanoids, precursors to prostaglandins (PG), leukotrienes (LT), and thromboxanes (TX). These molecules, the PG and TX, for example, have actions similar to hormones but there is a key distinction between them and hormones. By definition, a hormone is a compound that is made in one organ in the body but travels and acts on tissues elsewhere in the body. The difference here is that PG and TX don't travel; they act in the cells where they are synthesized.

Can omega-3 by synthesized from omega-6?

No. They do not convert from one to another.

On Preventable Causes of Death

In a recent assessment of 12 diet and life-style factors and preventable causes of death using US national health statistics, second to high salt intake (associated with an estimated average of 102,000 deaths per year), low intake of EPA and DHA omega-3 fatty acids were attributed with an estimated average of 84,000 deaths per year by heart attack or stroke. High intake of trans fats was attributed with the next greatest risk at 82,000 deaths. High blood pressure and tobacco use were attributed with the most deaths*.

---

* Danaei G, et al. The preventable causes of death in the United States: Comparative risk assessment of dietary, lifestyle, and metabolic risk factors. *PLoS (Public Library of Science) Medicine,* 2009;6:1-23.

ENDNOTES

1   Farzaneh-Far R, et al. Association of marine omega-3 fatty acid levels with telomeric aging in patients with coronary heart disease. *J Am Medical Assoc* 2010;303(3):250-257.

2   Harris WS, et al. Towards establishing dietary reference intakes for eicosapentaenoic and docosahexaenoic acids. *J Nutr* 2009;139:804S-819S.

3   Brenna JT, et al. Alpha-linolenic acid supplementation and conversion to n-3 long-chain polyunsaturated fatty acids in humans. *Prostaglandins Leukotr Essent Fatty Acids* 2009;80:85-91.

4   Harris WS, et al. Stearidonic acid-enriched soybean oil increased the omega-3 index, an emerging cardiovascular risk marker. *Lipids* 2008;43(9):805-811.

5   Lemke SL, et al. Dietary intake of stearidonic acid–enriched soybean oil increases the omega-3 index: Randomized, double-blind clinical study of efficacy and safety. *A J Clin Nutr* 2010;92:766-75.

6   Gropper SS, et al. *Advanced Nutrition and Human Metabolism* (5th ed.). Belmont, CA. Wadsworth/Cengage Learning, 2009.

7   Calder P. n-3 polyunsaturated fatty acids, inflammation, and inflammatory diseases. *A J Clin Nutr* 2006;83:1505S-1519S.

8   Innis SM. Dietary omega-3 fatty acids and the developing brain. *Brain Res* 2008;1237:35-43.

9   Lauritzen L, et al. The essentiality of long chain n-3 fatty acids in relation to development and function of the brain and retina. *Progress Lipid Res* 2001;40:1-94.

10 Hibbeln JR. Depression, suicide and deficiencies of omega–3 essential fatty acids in modern diets. In Simopoulos AP, Bazan

NG, eds., *Omega-3 Fatty Acids, the Brain and Retina.World Rev Nutr Diet*, pp. 17-30. Karger: Basil, Switzerland, 2009.

11 Carlson SE. Early determinants of development: A lipid perspective. *Am J Clin Nutr* 2009:89:1523S-1529S.

12 Uauy R, et al. Essential fatty acids in visual and brain development. *Lipids* 2001; 36(9):885-895.

13 Serhan CN, et al. Anti-inflammatory and proresolving lipid mediators. *Ann Rev Pathol Mech Dis* 2008;3:279-312.

14 Institute of Medicine. Dietary reference intakes for energy, carbohydrate, fiber, fat, fatty acids, cholesterol, protein, and amino acids. National Academy of Sciences: Washington, DC, 2002.

15 National Library of Medicine, Agency for Healthcare Research & Quality Evidence Report No. 93 (AHRQ, 2004) url: http://www.ncbi.nlm.nih.gov/books/bv.fcgi?rid=hstat1a.table.35384

16 Harris WS. The Omega-3 Index: Clinical utility for therapeutic intervention. *Curr Cardiol Rep* 2010; 12:503-508.

17 Omega-3 absorption pilot trial, unpublished data. Portland, Oregon, 2010.

18 Harris WS, et al. Omega-6 fatty acids and risk for cardiovascular disease. *Circulation* 2009;119: 902-907.

19 Hibbeln JR, et al. Healthy intakes of n-3 and n-6 fatty acids: Estimations considering worldwide diversity. *Am J Clin Nutr* 2006; 83:1483S-1493S.

20 Hibbeln JR, et al. Increasing homicide rates and linoleic acid consumption among five western countries, 1961–2000. *Lipids* 2004;39(12):1207-1213.

21 Department of Health and Human Services. Substances Affirmed as Generally Recognized as Safe: Menhaden oil. 21 CFR Part 184. Food and Drug Administration. Federal Register, 1997; 62 (108): 30751-30757.

22   Jellin, JM, et al. Pharmacist's Letter/Prescriber's Letter Natural Medicine Comprehensive Database. Stockton, CA: Therapeutic Research Faculty, 2011.

23   Harris WS. Expert opinion: Omega-3 fatty acids and bleeding: Cause for concern? *Am J Cardiol* 2007;99:44C-46C.

24   Martin JG. EPA but not DHA appears to be responsible for the efficacy of omega-3 long chain polyunsaturated fatty acid supplementation in depression: Evidence from a meta-analysis of randomized controlled trials. *J Am Coll Nutr* 2009;28(5):525-542.

25   Appleton KM, et al. Updated systematic review and meta-analysis of the effects of n-3 long-chain polyunsaturated fatty acids on depressed mood. *Am J Clin Nutr* 2010;91:757-770.

26   Goldberg RJ, Katz J. A meta-analysis of the analgesic effects of omega-3 polyunsaturated fatty acid supplementation for inflammatory joint pain. *Pain* 2007;129(1-2):210-223.

27   Muldoon MF, et al. Serum phospholipid docosahexaenonic acid is associated with cognitive functioning during middle adulthood. *J Nutr* 2010;140(4):848-853.

28   Whalley LJ, et al. Cognitive aging, childhood intelligence, and the use of food supplements: Possible involvement of n-3 fatty acids. *Am J Clin Nutr* 2004;80:1650-1657.

29   Personal communication. Doug Bibus, 2010.

30   Albert CM, et al. Blood levels of long-chain n-3 fatty acids and the risk of sudden death. *N Engl J Med* 2002;346:1113-1118.

31   Itomura M, et al. Factors influencing EPA+DHA levels in red blood cells in Japan. *In Vivo* 2008;22 (1):131-135.

32   Harris WS, von Schacky C. The Omega-3 Index: A new risk factor for death from coronary heart disease? *Prev Med* 2004;39:212-220.

33   Dyerberg J, et al. Fatty acid composition of the plasma lipids in Greenland Eskimos. *Am J Clin Nutr* 1975;28(9):958-966.

NOTES

CHAPTER 2

Getting Omega-3 from Foods

THE BASICS

Fish: The best direct sources of omega-3s

Fish and seafood are the richest, natural sources of DHA and EPA omega-3s. Fatty fish from the deep sea and other cold waters contain the most DHA and EPA. Fish carry omega-3 fatty acids in their body fat. EPA and DHA do not solidify at cold temperatures and allow the fish to exist in the cold waters. The colder the water, the greater the amount of EPA and DHA in the fish; this is a result of natural evolution. Dietary supplements and foods fortified with DHA and EPA are additional direct sources.

Plants: Indirect sources of omega-3s

Some plants, such as flax seed, chia seed, and soybeans contain omega-3s. However, they do not contain EPA and DHA, the long-chain omega-3s (EPA and DHA are called *biofunctional* because they have a direct impact on the body).

Instead, these plant sources provide ALA, a short-chain omega-3 that must undergo metabolic conversion to EPA in the body. Unfortunately, clinical research has confirmed that this conversion is poor in most humans (only 5-10% of the ALA is converted to EPA on average)[1]. This means that most of us need to ingest roughly 20 times the amount of fatty acids from the plant foods to get the equivalent EPA in a serving of fish. In addition, through conversion, these plant sources provide only a negligible amount of DHA (less than 0.5% conversion)[2]. So it's difficult to get adequate amounts of both EPA and DHA from plants alone. (See more about plant sources below, including information on algal sources and SDA.)

The simplest way to get what you need

The simplest and most cost-effective way to ensure regular, adequate intake of EPA and DHA for healthy individuals is to consume oily fish, such as tuna, sardines, or salmon, twice a week. Good choices would be a tuna sandwich or sardines with crackers for lunch once a week and fish for dinner once a week. For general nutrition, experts recommend 250–500 milligrams of DHA and EPA per day, or eating fish a couple times a week.

Table 2-1 DHA and EPA Content in Commonly Consumed Fish*†

Fish	EPA (mg)	DHA (mg)	Total
Chinook salmon	858	618	1476
Bluefin tuna	310	970	1280
Pink salmon	450	630	1080
Sockeye salmon	450	595	1045
Rainbow trout	284	697	981
Sardines (canned)	400	433	833
Albacore tuna (canned in water)	198	535	733
Sea bass	175	473	648
Halibut	77	318	395
Light tuna (canned in water)	40	190	230
Grouper	30	180	210
Haddock	65	138	203
Atlantic cod	0	130	130
Tilapia	4	110	114

Source: USDA Nutrient Data Lab.

*Per 3-ounce serving of fish cooked with dry heat.

†Presented in descending order of total EPA and DHA per serving

Why weekly intake may be enough

EPA and DHA are fat-soluble nutrients that can be stored in blood and tissue. Intake over the course of days and weeks is what matters to those blood and tissue levels for the omega-3s to do their work in the body.

Table 2-2 Forms of Omega-3 and Their Sources

Form of omega-3	Plant foods	Marine foods	Fortified foods	Dietary supplements
ALA	Yes		Yes	Yes
SDA	Yes		Yes	
EPA		Yes	Yes	Yes
DPA		Yes		Yes
DHA		Yes	Yes	Yes

MORE ABOUT MARINE SOURCES

How much fish is recommended?

For a healthy individual, an average daily intake of at least 250 mg of EPA and DHA (combined) is the amount shown to reduce risk of heart disease, including sudden cardiac death (note that 500 mg EPA and DHA daily is preferred). An average daily target of 250 mg of EPA and DHA can easily be consumed by eating fish once or twice a week, depending on the fish. For example, one 4-ounce serving of fresh Chinook salmon OR one 5-ounce serving of canned pink salmon in a week would deliver this!

The American Dietetic Association, American Heart Association, and American Psychiatric Association have recommended that adults eat fish two or more times a week. There are no formal recommendations for children but experts recommend they follow adult guidelines[3,4,5,6,7].

Fish vs. supplements

Fish is an important source of protein and trace minerals as well as EPA and DHA omega-3. If clients are amenable, consuming omega-3s is best done through foods. Fish can be easily incorporated into the regular meal program for individuals or families and can displace other, less nutritious food choices. Omega-3 capsules supply only omega-3, and like all supplements, benefitting from them requires buying them and establishing habits to take them. However, recommending food or supplements depends on the client's preferences, their health, their food habits, and their willingness to incorporate something new.

> ### Research Findings
> Compared to individuals who consume little or no seafood, those who consume a modest amount of omega-3s (250-500 mg of EPA + DHA/d, or 1-2 servings of oily fish/week) have a 25-50% lower risk for CHD death*.
>
> ---
> * Mozaffarian D. Fish and n-3 fatty acids for the prevention of fatal coronary heart disease and sudden cardiac death. A J Clin Nutr 2008; 87:1991S-1996S.

> ### Are EPA and DHA destroyed by cooking?
> Surprisingly, EPA and DHA are more stable in cooking than you might expect. There is some loss, depending how the food is prepared. When fish is cooked quickly at a high temperature, most of the EPA and DHA are retained.

Tips for helping parents help their children eat fish

- Let parents know that children usually need to see a new food 6 or more times before they accept it and that it's best to serve new foods with familiar foods. Serving a small amount of a new food without expecting it to be accepted the first few times is a good plan. Observing other family members enjoying a food encourages children. If the parents don't eat or enjoy fish, it's likely their children will follow that example, so parents may want to overcome their own reluctance.

- Encourage parents to be creative about incorporating fish into weekly meals, perhaps in casseroles, soups, or salads. Both canned tuna and salmon work in many dishes as meat substitutes. Fresh fish served off the grill can be more appealing as a special meal; canned tuna mixed with pickles or veggies is a favorite among older children. Exploring toddlers will often eat fish (if fresh, carefully remove bones).

- Recommend eggs with EPA and DHA (see below).

- Dietary supplements are a good option but be sure to guide the parents on label reading so that they receive adequate amounts of DHA and EPA for the price (see Chapter 3 on dietary supplements).

- Remind parents that their child will double or triple in size between age of 4 and 10 years, and there is significant demand for essential fat nutrition to support this growth. Encouraging healthy food habits is a lifelong gift to a child.

Canned vs. fresh fish

EPA and DHA are in the oily part of the fish and are retained in both fresh and canned fish. However, there is more EPA and DHA in fish canned in water than in oil because the omega-3 stays in the fish rather than leaching out into the vegetable oil that it is packed in. Note: Fish canned in oil is *not* packed in fish oil; it is packed in vegetable oil.

Fast-food fish

As with most nutritional counseling advice, fast foods and processed foods are low on the list of recommended foods for good nutrition. The type of fish commonly used by fast food restaurants in a fish sandwich is low in EPA and DHA omega-3. A breaded and deep-fried fish patty yields about 100 mg EPA and DHA or less and contains considerable additional fat used in preparation.

Similarly, breaded fish sticks may provide a small amount of long-chain omega-3s, but the amount is insufficient to meet the levels recommended by experts for growing children. Label reading is important. Some companies selling fish sticks don't claim to provide any EPA and DHA omega-3, again, because the fish they use is very low in omega-3. (Perhaps we should ask ourselves whether fish sticks that don't provide EPA and DHA should be considered fish?) One company selling breaded fish sticks advertises that it contains 32 mg EPA and DHA omega-3 in each 3-ounce serving (6 sticks). That said, fast food choices may be better than no fish at all, and they could serve as an introduction to eating fish for children. Lest we forget, 3 ounces of light tuna contains 230 mg of EPA and DHA, albacore tuna supplies 730 mg, and pink salmon (available in box stores) provides more than 1000 mg EPA and DHA in each 3-ounce serving. A one- or two-ounce serving of these foods can deliver powerful nutrition to a child.

MORE ABOUT PLANT SOURCES
Flax seeds

Flax seeds are small, light brown, oval seeds with a slightly nutty flavor and smell. Flax seeds are an excellent source of ALA (the short-chain omega-3) and good sources of protein (about 20%) and fiber, both soluble and insoluble (about 28%). Flax is also a good source of lignans (phytoestrogens), other phytonutrients, and antioxidants. Like most seeds and nuts, it is gluten-free. The seeds are about 42% fat (by weight), of which about 57% is ALA omega-3. For reference, a tablespoon (7 grams) of ground flax seed contains about 1500 mg ALA omega-3.

> **Note on ALA conversion**
> While flax, chia, and hemp seeds are nutritious foods and sources of ALA omega-3, the conversion rate of ALA to EPA is low, and conversion to ALA to DHA is negligible.

Flax seed, whole or ground, and the oil pressed from flax seed are readily available on the market in both organic and conventional forms. Ground flax seed and oil are often added to blender drinks, and the oil can be used as salad dressing.

Note: Whole flax seed must be chewed thoroughly to get the nutritional value; otherwise, it is simply a whole seed fiber. Ground flax seeds and oil need to be kept away from oxygen and refrigerated. It's best not to cook with flax seed oil, though it can be added to dishes near the end of cooking and eaten immediately.

Chia seeds

Chia is the edible seeds of the desert plant *Salvia hispanica*. They are small round seeds with a slight nutty flavor and smell. Like flax seed, chia seed is a good source of ALA; they also contain about 15% protein and fiber, both soluble and insoluble fiber (about 40%). Chia seeds also contain minerals, such as calcium and magnesium, and are gluten-free. The seeds are about 30% fat (by weight), of which about 56% is ALA omega-3. For example, a 7 gram serving of chia seed contains about 1200 mg ALA omega-3. Organic and conventional chia seeds are becoming more popular for use in cereals and beverage.

Fruits and nuts

Avocados contain ALA omega-3 (an average avocado contains about 220 mg ALA). Among the nuts, walnuts are the highest source of ALA. A ¼ cup of chopped walnuts contains about 2500 mg of ALA omega-3.

Hemp seeds

Hemp (*Cannabis sativa*) has been cultivated for thousands of years, for both the fiber and seed. Hemp contains about equal amounts of protein, carbohydrates, and fat. It is a good source of fiber (about 30%) and also contains some B-vitamins and minerals (e.g., magnesium and manganese). The seeds are about 30% fat, of which 15–20% is ALA omega-3. Hemp is unique in that it is a source of two other polyunsaturated fatty acids: it contains 2-3 % gamma linolenic acid (GLA, omega-6) and up to 3% stearidonic acid (SDA, omega 3).

DHA from algae

DHA algal oil is a specially produced product for use in food fortification and dietary supplements. It is also used in infant formula. It is vegetarian, not genetically modified, and derived from algae. Both capsule and oil products are available on the market. See labels for DHA amounts. Note: The kelp used as a sushi wrap does not contain meaningful amounts of DHA.

SDA: A new plant form of omega-3

Stearidonic acid (SDA) omega-3 has been genetically modified into soybean oil although SDA does not naturally occur in soybean oil. It is approved for use in foods in North America. SDA-rich soybean oil will be marketed as a natural, sustainable plant form of omega-3 and has received Generally Regarded as Safe (GRAS) status in North America but not in Europe. Foods containing genetically modified SDA are labeled *SDA-rich soybean oil* on food packaging.

On the omega-3 metabolic pathway, SDA is one step closer than ALA to becoming EPA; hence, conversion of SDA to EPA is better than ALA to EPA. Conversion of SDA to EPA is about 17% in humans with no appreciable conversion to DHA[8,9]. SDA occurs naturally in echium oil, a largely unknown plant, and there is a small amount in hemp seed.

Canola oil as a source of omega-3

Compared to other vegetable and cooking oils, canola oil offers some advantages. It is low in saturated fat, contains about 60% monounsaturated fat omega-9, and contains more ALA than most vegetable oils (about 11% ALA).

Notably, it also contains considerably fewer omega-6 fats than corn, cottonseed, and soybean oils.

What about corn, soybean, and cottonseed oils?

These are important because nearly 90% of the ALA in our diet comes from fats and oils[10]. And while nearly all of the vegetable oil consumed in the United States is made from canola, corn, soybean, and cottonseed (all rich sources of omega-6 linoleic acid), only canola and soy offer a measurable amount of ALA. Of these two ALA contributors, canola supplies significantly fewer omega-6 fats. Note: Some vegetable oil manufacturers are using farming practices to reduce levels of ALA in order to extend shelf-life (as a polyunsaturated fat, ALA is subject to oxidation and rancidity). For example, soybean oil typically contains about 8% ALA, but low-ALA soybean oil used commercially contains 3-4%[10]. These modifications are not generally noted on labels.

Plant sources of omega-3 increase EPA but not DHA.

Increasing EPA levels in the body is useful. EPA omega-3 works in concert with ARA (arachidonic acid) omega-6 as eicosanoids. Eicosanoids (hormone-like compounds) are precursors to prostaglandins, thromboxanes, and leukotrienes which the body uses in managing many internal functions, including blood pressure, breathing, and inflammation. DHA functions in human metabolism and is also structurally important in some organs, such as the brain, eyes and gonads. Research is increasingly showing that EPA and DHA complement each other and several studies suggest they work better together than either alone.

Do vegetarians need less EPA and DHA?

All humans utilize EPA and DHA. It has been suggested that vegetarians, in the absence of fatty acids from meat and dairy products, may convert plant forms of omega-3 to EPA and DHA more efficiently; however, that has not been shown to be true. Furthermore, those who eat a plant-based diet often consume large amounts of omega-6 fatty acids, especially if they regularly consume soy-based and manu-factured vegetarian foods; that heavy con-sumption of omega-6 inhibits conversion of the plant forms to EPA and DHA. Healthy tissue levels of EPA and DHA are important for everyone.

FORTIFIED FOODS

Omega-3 eggs

Eggs naturally contain some DHA, about 25 mg in the yolk. They are often a good choice of protein and DHA for elders, moms, and young children.

Eggs fortified with omega-3s are readily available; they can provide short-chain ALA or long-chain EPA and DHA. Which omega-3 they provide depends on what the chickens are fed, usually flax seed or fish oil. The only way to know which omega-3 is in the egg is to read the label. Fortified eggs cost more than regular eggs so consider your clients' overall diet before making a recommendation. If they are fish-eaters or fish oil supplement consumers, it may not be worth the additional cost to buy fortified eggs.

Recommending foods fortified with omega-3s

Whether to recommend fortified foods depends on the individual or family. Your client may want the convenience of such foods. Consumers can obtain EPA and DHA directly from marine sources or delivered through supplements or added to familiar foods for convenience. However, the amount of EPA and DHA can vary from 20 mg to 2000 mg per serving in any of these sources so reading labels is crucial. Getting sufficient amounts of EPA and DHA into our clients on a regular basis is what matters.

All types of foods, from waters to bars, from cookies to spaghetti sauce, are now available fortified with omega-3s. When both EPA and DHA are present in a fortified food, it is usually from purified fish. When the food is fortified with DHA only, it is usually from algal DHA and is vegetarian. See Table 2-3 for more information.

When EPA and DHA occur together in fortified foods, such as orange juice, peanut butter, or chocolate, they are mostly likely sourced from purified fish oil, and minimizing any fish taste during this process is a challenge. In these instances, food manufacturers are appealing to convenience and familiarity to deliver essential nutrients, and as with eggs, it comes at a higher price.

Soybeans, of course, are a plant food and naturally contain ALA, the short-chain omega-3, so when DHA appears in soy milk, it has been added, usually from the algal source. **Note:** The amount of omega-3 claimed on the soymilk package may be the combined total of ALA from the soybeans and the added DHA.

As always, reading the label is key. If you want your client to get more EPA, then a DHA-fortified orange juice isn't the answer. Note: Read the allergen statement on the food label. If it states *does not contain fish*, then any EPA or DHA in the product is not from fish. Often, but not always,

Table 2-3 Commonly Used Omega-3 Forms and Sources in Fortified Foods

Form of omega-3	Commonly used sources
Short-chain omega-3	
ALA	Flax seed, soybean, or canola oil
SDA	GM* soybean oil
Long-chain omega-3	
EPA	Purified fish oil
DHA	Purified fish oil or algal oil

*GM = Genetically Modified

a plant-based food, such as soy milk or cereal, will contain a plant-sourced (short-chain) omega-3.

Omega-3 in beverages

Because EPA and DHA are long-chain fatty acids, they are by nature insoluble in water. Nonetheless, there is a desire by food manufacturers to get EPA and DHA into water and sodas. One such water beverage is already on the market; it claims to provide a small amount of EPA and DHA in water with no calories. At this writing, the absorbability of EPA and DHA in water, consumed away from food, has not been tested and confirmed. Fortifying fruit juices with EPA and DHA and adding algal DHA to soymilk isn't new. Clients may find these products helpful.

Omega-3s in snack foods

Many of the snack foods on the market, such as tortilla chips and granola bars, contain ALA omega-3. There is a current trend to add ground, plant-sourced omega-3 to foods in order to claim the omega-3 is there; however, the amount, even in multiple servings, is insignificant. Companies can claim that a nutrient is present without stating an amount per serving. Have you noticed that mayonnaise now advertises that it is a source of omega-3? That's because the soybean oil contains ALA; there may be minimal DHA if real egg yolk is used.

Here's a tip: Read the ingredient label. If ground flax powder is the last ingredient listed, then the snack food could be a negligible source of any omega-3. On the other hand, fortified snack foods can provide a reasonable amount of EPA and DHA per serving. In general, the amount of EPA and DHA in common snack foods ranges from 30–100 mg per serving. There is a snack bar currently on the market that contains 300 mg EPA and DHA, and a functional food meal bar that provides a generous 2000 mg EPA and DHA per serving.

Consuming omega-3s in snack foods can be an added benefit and practical when traveling although fish consumption and/or supplements may be more reliable options.

Quality of EPA and DHA in fortified foods

The sources of EPA and DHA used in our food supply are purified. The fish, usually anchovies, are sustainably caught, refined, purified, and powdered, then added to foods. Much of the effort in manufacturing these very-long-chain fatty acids is in preventing oxidation and degradation and then incorporating them into packaged foods while managing the issues of taste, dose, and stability. This is food science at its best. Shipping and storage temperature and shelf-life are considered as well.

Cooking with fish oil

Using fish oil in heat-prepared foods is *not* a good idea. The long-chain, unsaturated fatty acids will oxidize readily, particularly in open exposure to oxygen. However, using some fresh cod liver oil or fish oil in a salad dressing or refrigerated dip is a tasty idea. This is fine when the food is consumed immediately.

> **Tip on Reading labels**
>
> If a fortified food label claims that it contains omega-3, you can generally assume that it contains the short-chain omega-3. Foods fortified with EPA and DHA generally indicate that on the label, though not always.

> # Keep it simple.
>
> Increasing overall tissue levels of EPA and DHA will reduce risk for chronic disease.

FREQUENTLY ASKED QUESTIONS

Fat is still fat! Some of my clients follow a very low-fat food program

Yes, omega-3 is a fat and it provides 9 calories per gram, just like other fats. However, omega-3s are an important source of healthy fat in the diet. Both omega-3 and omega-6 fats are called dietary *essential* fats because humans require them and cannot synthesize them. They are indispensable polyunsaturated fatty acids, which, under normal circumstances, are not used as a fuel or a calorie source by the body but rather serve other functions. They are innately different from monounsaturated and saturated fats.

How do I advise my vegan and vegetarian clients?

The most practical approach is to advise regular and sufficient consumption of plant-based omega-3.

- 1 tablespoon of flaxseed *oil* will provide, after conversion, about 350–400 mg of EPA; 2 tablespoons of milled or ground flaxseed will provide about 150 mg EPA, if one assumes a 5% conversion rate of ALA to EPA.
- Flax seed oil, ground flax, and chia seeds can be added to blender drinks and used in baked products.
- To ensure intake of DHA, include regular consumption of a supplement containing vegetarian (algal) DHA available in vegetarian capsules or a fortified food.
- Recommend use of canola oil in the kitchen.
- Limit plant sources that are high in omega-6 fatty acids, such as soy, corn, and sunflower oil, as these

can inhibit conversion of ALA to the longer chain omega-3s.

- Nuts such as walnuts also provide ALA and are also great sources of fiber and high quality proteins as are flax and chia seeds.
- Other options are genetically modified EPA in supplement form.

> Sufficient intake of DHA during pregnancy benefits mother and child. Pregnant women who follow vegan diets have some of the lowest levels of DHA in the world[*,**].
>
> ---
> * Hibbeln, JD, *Prostaglandins, Leukotrienes & Essent Fatty Acids* 2009;81:179-186.
> **Personal communication, SE Carlson, 2008.

We've polluted the ocean, so isn't fish to be avoided?

Fish is a viable and valuable food source. However, some fish are best avoided or eaten infrequently, for example, shark, swordfish, and sturgeon. These fish, as well as other predator fish that live a long time, have longer exposure to pollutants. In part, this is what makes short-lived fish such as sardines and trout good dietary choices. Fish caught in large open seas, such as albacore tuna from North America,

---

Risk vs. Benefit

"<u>Conclusion</u>: For major health outcomes among adults, based on *both* the strength of the evidence and the potential magnitudes of effect, the benefits of fish intake exceed the *potential* risks. For women of childbearing age, benefits of modest fish intake, excepting a few selected species, also outweigh risks [emphasis added]*."

---

* [1]Mozaffarian D, Rimm EB. Evaluating the risks and the benefits fish intake, contaminants, and human health. *JAMA* 2006;296(15):1885.

---

salmon from Alaska, and farmed rainbow trout are also excellent sources of protein and omega-3s with low levels of mercury and dioxins.

The Monterey Bay Aquarium Seafood Watch® program rates fish and seafood by environmental impact. They recently added a Super Green List, which considers both environmental impact and toxin exposure. Their website is user-friendly http://www.montereybayaquarium.org/cr/seafoodwatch.aspx. The Environmental Defense Fund (www.edf.org) is another good resource for learning about fish and the environment.

Aren't we depleting the fish in the sea?

The Marine Stewardship Council is a global, non-profit

organization working to safeguard and sustain the world's seafood supply. Their vision is a world in which the oceans are teeming with life, providing seafood for current and future generations. They are independent and do not certify fisheries; they have a third-party certification based on standards. They work with wild caught fish, not farmed. Fish and seafood that meets their standards will have a MSC ecolabel™. You can advise clients to look for this in grocery stores and restaurants. There is a link on their website to locate local MSC certified foods. (www.msc.org)

What if I choose not to recommend fish to my clients or what if my client refuses to eat fish?

Consider how to guide your clients to incorporate EPA and DHA into their diet from other sources, such as fortified foods and dietary supplements. Remind them that EPA and DHA are the most biofunctional omega-3s and are required for optimal health. Regular consumption of EPA and DHA is linked to primary prevention of heart disease.

What about my clients who are allergic to fish?

First, it is important to identify the allergy as clearly as possible. Some people are allergic to shellfish but not finfish, and vice versa. Because allergens exist in the protein constituent, it is best to avoid the offending foods. However, there are some fish-allergic individuals who can take purified fish oil capsules when the oil is purified to a non-detectable level of proteins; this is the case with better-quality products and can be verified through independent testing.

What's more, some individuals who are allergic to fish can consume traditionally processed cod liver oil and here

On Fish, Pregnancy, and Our Future Generations

In 2004, the US Food and Drug Administration (FDA) and the Environmental Protection Agency (EPA) published advice for pregnant women and young children that said to avoid four specific fish (shark, swordfish, king mackerel, and tilefish) and to limit fish and seafood to 12 ounces or less per week. The reason for limiting fish intake were concerns about the risk for mercury exposure. However, steps to ensure sufficient intake of EPA and DHA omega-3 for mom and developing infant were not outlined, and fish consumption declines*, understandably, following national advisories.

A landmark study published in *The Lancet* in February 2007** reported results of a study that assessed the diet of nearly 12,000 pregnant women and the developmental, behavioral, and cognitive processes of their children from 6 months to 8 years of age. The children born of women who followed the equivalent of the US FDA's and EPA's advice were associated with an increased risk of being in the lowest quartile for development of verbal IQ. These children also had a higher risk of suboptimal development of social, communication, and fine motor skills when their mothers consumed less than 12 ounces of fish or seafood while pregnant. This study was carefully controlled for 28 potential confounding variables, including education, ethnicity, housing, partnership, alcohol and tobacco use, and 12 food groups in addition to fish.

Beliefs and media reports around fish consumption are complex, but insufficient intake of essential omega-3 fatty acids during pregnancy has long-lasting and detrimental effects on the development of our youth.

---

* Oken E, Kleinman KP, et al. Decline in fish consumption among pregnant women after a national mercury advisory. *Obstet Gynecol* 2003;102:346-351.
**Hibbeln JR, Davis JM, et al. Maternal seafood consumption in pregnancy and neurodevelopmental outcomes in childhood (ALSPAC study): An observational cohort study. *Lancet*, 2007; 369:578-585.

is why: if the liver is cut cleanly from the cod fish, it does not come in contact with the fish body muscle which may be the source of the allergen; if this is the case, then oil pressed from the liver will not contain the allergen.

Navigating your client through this will require collaboration and testing with an allergist. Remember, EPA and DHA are involved in immune function.

What do I tell my pregnant clients about eating fish during their pregnancy?

DHA is directly involved with fetal development (brain, eyes, nerve, and immune systems) and the mother is the sole source for the infant. If the mom is not consuming DHA omega-3 while pregnant, the DHA in her body will be used and depleted. Most pregnant women in North America severely *under*-consume DHA. Experts recommend a minimum daily intake of 200–300 mg DHA, and some suggest 900 mg/d to cover the needs of both infant and mother. Current mean intakes of DHA during pregnancy range between 70–80 mg/d. In one study, 90% of the pregnant women were consuming less than 300 mg/d.

Help your pregnant clients create a plan to regularly consume EPA and DHA omega-3 from foods or supplements. More than 1000 mg of DHA has been safely used in clinical trials with pregnant women[11,12,13,4].

What is the best value-for-the-dollar for my clients?

Regularly eating canned tuna, salmon, or sardines is the most economical way to go. Albacore (solid white) tuna has more than 3 times the amount of EPA and DHA as light tuna, and water-packed is the better choice. If, for example, you want your client to consume 250 mg EPA and DHA per day, they can do this by eating two cans of solid white tuna or sardines or salmon a week for a cost of less than a dollar a day.

Table 2-4: Best Fish Sources of EPA and DHA

Highest levels
Salmon
Anchovies
Bluefin tuna
Herring
Sardines

Lowest levels
Tilapia
Orange Roughy
Cod
Catfish
Haddock

Some foods have 32 mg DHA per serving and claim to be an "excellent source" of DHA

The 32 mg on the food label is calculated by considering 20% of the Daily Value of the Adequate Intake (AI) level for ALA as DHA at 10%. It's unusual for a claim to be allowed for nutrients on which only an AI level is established, and in this case, the AI is for ALA omega-3, not EPA and DHA. Sound confusing? It is, but the claim is currently allowed; it may be repealed. Most experts would like to see an RDA for EPA and DHA set at a minimum of 250 mg per day, making 32 mg a minimal amount for adults.

Is it worth incorporating omega-3 into my clients' weight-loss program?

In pilot research studies, when middle-aged adults added exercise and fish oil vs. placebo to their program, those who exercised and consumed fish oil lost the most body fat. Eating healthful fat aided fat loss. Scientists don't believe that EPA and DHA increase metabolism per se, but there is good reason to believe they improve metabolic efficiency. Achieving good nutrition status is also always helpful.

ENDNOTES

1   Harris WS, et al. Towards establishing dietary reference intakes for eicosapentaenoic and docosahexaenoic acids. *J Nutr* 2009;139:804S-819S.

2   Brenna JT, et al. Alpha-linolenic acid supplementation and conversion to n-3 long-chain polyunsaturated fatty acids in humans. *Prostaglandins, Leukotrienes & Essent Fatty Acids* 2009;80:85-91.

3   Mozaffarian D. Fish and n-fatty acids for the prevention of fatal coronary heart disease and sudden cardiac death. *A J Clin Nutr* 2008;87:1991S-1996S.

4   Kris-Etherton PM, et a. for the American Heart Association Nutrition Committee. Omega-3 fatty acids and cardiovascular disease: New recommendations from the American Heart Association. *Arteriosclerosis Thrombosis Vasc Biol* 2003; 23:151-152.

5   Freeman MP et al. Omega-3 fatty acids: Evidence base for treatment and future research in psychiatry. *J Clin Psychiatry* 2006; 67(12):1954-1967.

6   Kris-Etherton PM, Innis S. Position of the American Dietetic Association and Dietitians of Canada: Dietary fatty acids. J Am Dietetic Assn 2007;107:1599-1611.

7   Uauy R, Dangour AD. Fat and fatty acid requirements and recommendations for infants of 1-2 years and children of 2-18 years. *Ann Nutr & Metabol* 2009; 55:76- 96.

8   Harris WS, et al. Stearidonic acid-enriched soybean oil increased the omega-3 index, an emerging cardiovascular risk marker. *Lipids* 2008;43:805-811.

9   Lemke SL, et al. Dietary intake of stearidonic acid–enriched soybean oil increases the omega-3 index: Randomized,

double-blind clinical study of efficacy and safety. *A J Clin Nutr* 2010;92:766-775.

10 Kris-Etherton PM, et al. Polyunsaturated fatty acids in the food chain in the United States. *A J Clin Nutr* 2000:71(1):179S-188S.

11 Denomme J, et al. Directly quantitated dietary (n-3) fatty acid intakes of pregnant Canadian women are lower than current dietary recommendations. *J Nutr* 2005;135: 206-211.

12 Stark KD, et al. Comparison of bloodstream fatty acid composition from African-American women at gestation, delivery, and postpartum. *J Lipid Res* 2005;46:516-525.

13 Koletzko B, et al. The roles of long-chain polyunsaturated fatty acids in pregnancy, lactation and infancy: Review of current knowledge and consensus recommendations. *J Perinatal Med* 2008;36:5-14.

14 Hibbeln JR, Davis JM. Considerations regarding neuropsychiatric nutritional requirements for intakes of omega-3 highly unsaturated fatty acids. *Prostaglandins, Leukotrienes & Essent Fatty Acids* 2009;81:179-186.

NOTES

CHAPTER 3

Dietary Supplements

CHOOSING AND RECOMMENDING SUPPLEMENTS

Consuming omega-3s through the use of supplements is a safe and effective way to increase EPA and DHA levels, and current manufacturing processes by reputable companies mean that a pure, stable product reaches the client. Dietary supplements can be convenient but can also be more costly than incorporating fish into the diet, and they require establishing the practice of taking the supplements on a regular basis. Capsules that can be chewed or swallowed, candied-forms, and liquids are all available.

Dietary supplements that provide both EPA and DHA omega-3 are made from fish oil, cod liver oil, krill oil, salmon oil, and squid (calamari) oil (see Table 3-1). Fish oil comes from fatty fish; cod liver oil, as its name implies, comes from the processed livers of the cod fish. Krill oil is gaining

> Dietary supplements are a *supplement*, not a substitute, to the diet.

in popularity, both in consumption and for research. Krill oil contains EPA and DHA in phospholipid form and manufacturers of krill oil claim that this form is more bioavailable although this has not been confirmed. Humans readily absorb EPA and DHA from all of these marine sources.

Dietary supplements that provide DHA only are from algal sources, while dietary supplements that provide EPA only are from algal sources or genetically modified fungal sources. More genetically modified sources are being developed, largely due to the demand for EPA and DHA omega-3 and the concern with ocean supplies. A less commonly known omega-3, DPA is available from seal or menhaden oil. DPA is a metabolic intermediary between EPA and DHA that naturally occurs in seal blubber. Since Eskimos traditionally ate seal meat, there is increasing interest in learning more about this fatty acid; however, benefits beyond those proven for EPA and DHA are unknown at this time.

Because fish is a source of lean, complete protein and trace minerals, such as selenium, as well as EPA and DHA omega-3, eating fish on a regular basis is recommended. The American Dietetic Association, the American Heart Association, and the American Psychiatric Association recommend that adults eat fish two or more times a week[1,2,3].

MARINE SOURCES

Nearly all fish oil supplements sold in the US and Canada are made from sardines and anchovies, which are rich in

EPA and DHA omega-3. These small, short-lived fish are a good choice because they have little time in the ocean water for exposure to pollutants and metals. Even so, manufacturers purify the oil; that is, they remove saturated fats, contaminants, heavy metals, PCBs, etc. These small fish grow quickly, reproduce quickly, and are not endangered; and their harvesting does not compete with the food supply. The fleshy portion of the sardines and

Table 3-1 Sources of Long-Chain Omega-3s in Supplements

Source of EPA and DHA omega-3

- Fish oil (regular and concentrated)
- Cod liver oil
- Salmon oil
- Krill oil
- Squid (calamari) oil
- Menhaden oil

Source of DHA omega-3

- Algal oil

Source of EPA omega-3

- Algal oil
- Genetically-modified fungi

anchovies are used in animal feed, so none of the catch is wasted. Thus, they are a sustainable source.

Fish oil supplements from salmon oil have become popular, perhaps because consumers recognize salmon specifically as nutritious. They may also believe it is a better oil; it is a good source of omega-3s. The oil is pressed from the fish heads after the fillets and edible portions have been taken. Squid oil (also known as calamari oil) is also pressed from the head of the squid, after the edible portion is removed. For krill oil, the whole krill is pressed and that is why astanxanthin, the pigment that gives krill and salmon their pinkish color, is part of the krill oil capsules. The astanxanthin occurs as less than 1% of the oil.

The difference between fish oil and cod liver oil

Fish oil comes from the body of the fish source, e.g., anchovy or salmon. It is typically about 30% EPA and DHA omega-3, and the ratio of EPA and DHA varies by fish. Oil from the liver of cod (cod liver oil) is about 25% EPA and DHA, with relatively more DHA than EPA plus vitamins A and D (regular fish oil is not a natural source of vitamins A and D). The amount of vitamin A and D in the cod liver oil can vary by brand and here is why: when cod liver oil is refined, some of the vitamin A and D is removed along with the saturated fats. Brand marketing companies who sell cod liver oil will either add vitamins A and/or D back to the oil during bottling (e.g., 400 IU vitamin D3), or they will report an upper and lower range on the label reflecting seasonal variations in these vitamins. *Note on vitamin A:* Not all cod liver oil products contain high amounts of vitamin A. Manufacturers are aware of the concern with too much vitamin A, especially with pregnancy, and some have taken steps to reduce vitamin A levels. Be sure to read the label.

The first use of marine oils in medicine was reported in the 1700s, when giving cod liver oil to patients reduced symptoms of rheumatoid arthritis. In Scandinavian countries, cod liver oil has a long history of use in maternal and child health, and it is still common practice to feed cod liver oil to infants. Be forewarned: You will likely encounter older clients who were fed cod liver oil during their younger years and have negative associations with it, largely related to taste. Know that manufacturing practices have improved considerably and cod liver oil today doesn't taste anything like it did several decades ago. When fresh and kept refrigerated, it can be a cost-effective way to get a higher dose on a daily basis without swallowing pills. Many people report less burp or repeat with liquid cod liver oil. And when blended with juice or mixed into pudding, it can be quite pleasant.

Fish oil supplements may be blended with other nutrients

Most fish oil supplements sold on the market contain purified fish oil with an antioxidant added to prevent oxidation. Fish oil is also blended with omega-6 and omega-9 fatty acids and combining fish oil with other nutrients, usually for a specific health condition, has become more common. For example, products are available that combine fish oil with CoQ 10 for cardiovascular health or with chromium for people with diabetes. Adding vitamin D2 or D3 to fish oil is common. Be sure to read the label.

There are some advantages to combination products. They are convenient, they will reduce the number of bottles to buy, and they usually, but not always, reduce the number of capsules required to consume a particular dose. They may be a better value than buying individual bottles of products, but not always. Begin by identifying the appropriate dose of EPA and DHA for your client and then consider the strength of the evidence and potential benefit or barrier from adding additional nutrients. Consider these questions:

- Cost and compliance
  - ‣ If a combination product increases the monthly cost or the number of capsules required, will that reduce compliance?

- Sufficient dose and intended goal
  - ‣ Is the dose in the combination product sufficient to achieve the intended goal for supplementation? For example, the American Heart Association has specific recommendations for EPA and DHA to reduce triglycerides (See Resources). If the priority for your client is to reduce triglycerides but taking a combination product provides an insufficient dose, then consider recommending a concentrated fish oil product.
  - ‣ Is the dose of other ingredients (e.g., vitamin D) in the product adequate? Consider sources from other vitamin and mineral supplements, too.
- Form and compliance
  - ‣ Will recommending a flavored *liquid* fish oil product improve compliance? If so, then choose that over the combination capsule products.
- Availability
  - ‣ Is the combination product readily available for the client to purchase?

Consuming a sufficient dose is essential to achieving intended results. And always, making a daily task easier for your client improves compliance significantly.

ADVISING VEGAN AND VEGETARIAN CLIENTS

Plant-sources of omega-3 are shorter chain fatty acids that must be converted into the longer-chain EPA and DHA omega-3 for optimal benefit in the body (see Chapter 1). The best approach for vegan and vegetarian clients is a three-pronged one: 1) consume plenty of plant source omega-3 on a regular basis (e.g., 1 tablespoon of flax seed *oil* will provide about 350-400 mg EPA, after conversion); 2) consume a DHA supplement in vegetarian capsules or fortified food (e.g., juice); 3) use canola and olive oil instead of soybean or cottonseed oil in the kitchen.

Table 3-2 Forms of Available Supplements

- **Capsules:** range in size (from small to very large) and dose (from 200–700 mg EPA and DHA per capsule; read label).
    Tip: If one capsule contains 9 calories, then it contains 1 gram of oil. Most people consider this a large capsule.
- **Chewable:** flavored fish oil or sugar-based candies
- **Liquids:** flavored or unflavored oils
- **Pudding-like emulsions:** available in single-serving packets and bottles
- **Specialty food products**

ANTIOXIDANTS AND OTHER DETAILS ABOUT FISH OIL SUPPLEMENTS

Date of expiration

Marine oil supplements should have a date of expiration on the bottle; it is usually 3 years from the date of manufacture.

Antioxidants

Marine oil supplements should contain an antioxidant. These act as natural preservatives; they help stabilize the oil and keep it fresh during its shelf life. Vitamin E is the most commonly used antioxidant, although rosemary extract and ascorbyl palmitate (fat-soluble vitamin C) are also used.

Vitamin E

The amount of vitamin E added to fish oil can vary from a small amount intended to function only as an antioxidant to a larger amount intended to also provide nutritional value. You can discern how vitamin E is being used by reading the label. If vitamin E is included in the Other Ingredients listing and not declared in the Supplement Facts panel, then its purpose is to protect the oil from oxidation; if it's included in the Supplement Facts panel, then it will contribute to the daily intake. The amount can vary by company.

The Daily Value for vitamin E for adults and children over the age of 4 years is 30 IU. Different forms of vitamin E (e.g., alpha, gamma, or beta tocopherol) are used in fish oils because different forms offer different antioxidant capacities. They may be listed individually or as "mixed tocopherols." Note that only alpha tocopherol can be declared as vitamin E on the label. Also note that the natural form of vitamin E is *d*-alpha tocopherol, while the synthetic form of vitamin E is *dl*-alpha tocopherol. Both function as antioxidants.

Nearly all the natural vitamin E used in dietary supplements comes from highly refined soybean oil. As such, brand marketers cannot list the product as being free of soy and this has limitations for customers who are looking for soy-free products.

Other antioxidants

Rosemary extract has good antioxidant properties and is soy-free, but vitamin E is usually also added for best effectiveness. Ascorbyl palmitate is also used as an antioxidant but less often and usually as part of an antioxidant blend. Some companies are using other botanical extracts as stabilizers, such as oregano oil; again, they are usually part of an antioxidant blend.

Better fish oil manufacturers are constantly evaluating how to improve stability.

Emulsifiers

Emulsifiers are used when fish oil is blended, usually with non-fat-soluble nutrients. For example, when vitamin D or CoQ10 are added to the oil, an emulsifier may or may not be used because these are fat-soluble nutrients. When other nutrients (e.g., carnitine) are added to the oil, an emulsifier is used. The emulsifier most commonly used is soy lecithin and this again prevents a soy-free claim on the label.

About capsules

Regular fish oil capsules

Regular fish oil capsules are composed of gelatin, glycerin, and water. They are clear and can be swallowed or chewed. Unless stated, the gelatin is animal-sourced. Vegetarian capsules are available and will be so indicated on the label.

Enteric-coated capsules

An enteric-coated capsule is a capsule that has been coated so that it is resistant to gastric acids and thus releases lower in the gastrointestinal tract where the pH is higher. Enteric-coated capsules that contain fish oil are usually dark in color, but not all enteric-coated capsules are dark. Claims by companies who sell fish oil in enteric-coated capsules include the following: protecting the capsules from light and oxidation, reducing repeat or burping, and improving digestion.

Enteric-coated fish oil capsules generally cost more. They may protect the capsule contents from oxidation if the capsules are exposed (left out of the bottle), and there is some evidence that enteric-coating reduces burping but to date, there is no published evidence that the coating improves digestion in healthy humans. In fact, a pilot trial showed significantly better absorption from regular fish oil capsules when compared to enteric-coated capsules, though absorption from both was good[4].

Dark-colored capsules

Dark-colored capsules are used when fish oil is blended with other nutrients in order to hide the capsule contents, sometimes an emulsified slurry. Dark capsules are not necessarily enteric-coated. The coatings are food grade, such as carmine or caramel, and some coatings provide additional protection, such as titanium dioxide, a natural sunblock.

Table 3-3 What to Look For in an EPA and DHA Supplement

- Number of capsules or amount of liquid per serving
- Amount of EPA and DHA per serving
- Stored in an air-tight and opaque bottle
- Date of expiration
- Presence of antioxidants (e.g., vitamin E)
- Presence of allergens (e.g., soy)
- Price per dose
- Calories and sugar content, when sugar is added
- Storage requirements (e.g., liquids must be refrigerated)
- Presence of other nutrients and their relevance for client
- Source: natural, vegetarian, or genetically modified
- Independent testing of finished product

BEHIND THE FISH OIL CURTAIN

There are fish oil manufacturers and there are fish oil brand marketers. Fish oil manufacturers catch the fish, press the oil, and refine it; then they sell it to brand marketing companies, who encapsulate or bottle the oil, put their label on it, market it, distribute it, and sell it.

Manufacturing

Several steps are taken to purify the oil in the refining process. In very large containers, the oil is first filtered, which removes proteins and saturated fats, then purified to remove heavy metals, such as mercury and lead, and organic compounds that occur in the ocean waters, such as polychlorinated biphenyls (PCBs) and dioxins. During this process, it is critical to protect the fragile, long-chain fatty acids from oxidation because they are easily oxidized. In fact, time, temperature, and use of antioxidants are critical elements in the manufacturing and lead to quality differences in the finished product. For example, fast production and exposure to high temperatures can strip the oil, increase oxidation, and lead to faster degradation. Finally, processing the oil, transporting the oil, and encapsulating the oil at low temperatures and in the absence of oxygen (by flushing with nitrogen gas, called a *nitrogen flush*) are critical for maintaining freshness and preventing oxidized (rancid) oil.

Quality standards for processing fish oil are critical, and there are maximum measures for purity and oxidation. The international standard for manufacturing omega-3 from fish was developed in 2002 and updated in 2006. The monograph outlining this standard is known as the

GOED (Global Organization of EPA and DHA Omega-3) Voluntary Monograph and was the first of its kind to establish limits for heavy metals, PCBs, dioxins, and freshness measures for North America. The original monograph was developed by a group of omega-3 experts who saw the need for an international standard for analytical methods, quality, and purity standards. Compliance with these standards is currently voluntary. Companies who are members of the GOED sign an affidavit agreeing to meet the quality standards. Signing this affidavit is a requirement for membership. (For more information, see the summary of the GOED monograph in the Resources section or go to www.GOEDomega3.com)

Brand marketers, those companies that sell fish oil to retail stores and consumers, buy bulk fish oil from the manufacturers and have it put into capsules and bottled or have it bottled as liquid oil. At this step, antioxidants (e.g., vitamin E or rosemary oil) or flavors (e.g., citrus or strawberry) or other vitamins (e.g., vitamin D) can be added. Note that this creates differences between products available on the market. Some brand marketers also buy capsules already made and bottle those. Protecting the oil from oxidation during these processes, again, is critical.

After the products are labeled and sealed, the finished product is shipped to a warehouse and from there it is ready to ship to retail stores, direct to consumer, or direct to doctor or dietitian. The labels contain standardized information, including the name of the product, the company logo, the number of capsules, the Supplement Facts panel, ingredients, allergy statements, product claims, date of manufacture and/or expiration, and company contact information.

Examples of brand marketing companies include Barleans®, Nordic Naturals®, NatureMade®, and Carlsons®.

QUALITY DIFFERENCES IN FISH AND MARINE OIL SUPPLEMENTS

There are differences in the quality of marine oil products available on the market. Time for processing, temperature, handling, blending, exposure to oxygen, the presence or absence of antioxidants, and concentration all influence the integrity of the finished product.

Manufacturing, from the first press of the fish to the final bottling of the marine oil capsules, involves maintaining the nutrients and the quality of the oil while filtering and purifying the natural substance. In the making of better-quality marine oil supplements, steps must be taken to 1) *prevent oxidation* of the fresh oil while it 2) undergoes several stages of *filtration* and *purification* (necessary to meet quality standards) and 3) to *retain* the structurally sensitive EPA and DHA. All of this requires technical knowledge, advanced engineering, and skill. There is cost involved in retaining these naturally occurring nutrients through this complex process.

As with food manufacturing, faster processing, higher temperatures, and

> The very nature that makes EPA and DHA uniquely valuable for human nutrition (very long chains of highly unsaturated fatty acids/multiple double bonds) also makes it vulnerable to rancidity and destruction.

other short-cuts can be taken to save costs. For example, some manufacturers purify and test for every potential contaminate they can detect, while others do the minimum; some choose to comply with international standards for quality and others do not; some invest in human clinical research; and some (the leaders) are continually investing in improved technology while others are waiting for the results and will copy them (the followers). Choices made during manufacturing are reflected in the quality and cost of the finished product. Further, some fish oil manufacturers only produce premium oils and concentrates and others aim for higher volumes and low prices. There are large quality differences in what is available on the market.

Consider this analogy: both whole grain and white flour are, by definition, flour. They are both processed. One retains additional beneficial compounds inherent to the natural source (whole grain) and the other meets minimum standards (white). This is much the same with fish oil. All good fish oil products are refined, but they can be manufactured to meet minimum standards or they can be manufactured to meet those same standards *and* selectively retain qualities inherent to the original source (other fatty acids, more intact omega-3, etc).

PRODUCTION OF VEGETARIAN SUPPLEMENTS

Vegetarian sources that provide DHA from micro-algae are naturally sourced, then fermented in a contained, controlled environment.

READING THE LABEL

As mentioned earlier, reading the label is crucial for professionals and consumers alike. Not all omega-3 supplements are alike in what they offer and how they have been produced.

First look at the serving size, then the amount of EPA and DHA per serving. Do not confuse mg of fish oil with mg of EPA and DHA. Fish oil capsules can contain from 20%–70% EPA and DHA in each capsule.

On the example label below, each 2-capsule serving provides 600 mg EPA and DHA from 2400 mg of fish oil (two 1200 mg capsules is one serving). This product contains 25% omega-3.

Fish Oil Capsules		
1200 mg		
Supplement Facts		
Serving Size:	2 Softgels	
Servings Per Container:	60	
Amount per Serving		
Calories	25	
Calories from fat	21	
		% Daily Value
Total Fat	2.4 g	3%
Polyunsaturated fat	0.8 g	
Cholesterol	45 mg	15%
Vitamin E	3 IU	10%
Fish Oil		
EPA (mg)	360	
DHA (mg)	240	

In this example, it is common for clients to believe they are consuming 1200 mg of omega-3 from fish oil and they are not. Read the label for amount of EPA and DHA per serving. Dose matters. Further, a 1200-mg capsule is considered a large capsule so also consider compliance.

Product label claims

Thousands of human clinical trials have been published that show benefits with EPA and DHA omega-3, and the large percentage of these studies were done with subjects taking fish oil or consuming fish in the daily diet. Companies who sell dietary supplements are required to comply with the US FDA Dietary Supplement Health and Education Act of 1994 (21 CFR 101.93(g)).

In brief, companies are permitted to make claims that describe the effect of the supplement on the structure or function of the body but they are not permitted to claim that a product will cure, mitigate, treat, or prevent disease (these are known as *disease claims*). Dietary supplement companies are not required to show proof of efficacy before selling a product, although they are required to have substantiation for their claims and by law, the claims they make must be truthful and not misleading. In contrast, drug companies are required to have proof of efficacy before going to market and can make disease claims.

In reality, the quality of claims and strength of substantiation vary widely among brand marketers of fish oil and omega-3 supplements.

If you question a claim made by a brand marketer, simply contact the company and ask for their substantiation of the claim. They are required to have it available and

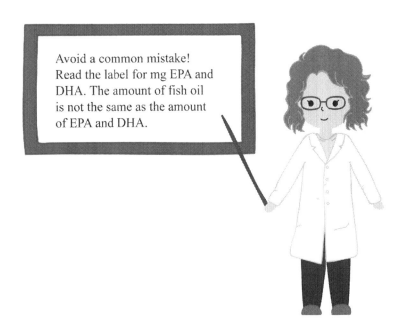

Avoid a common mistake!
Read the label for mg EPA and
DHA. The amount of fish oil
is not the same as the amount
of EPA and DHA.

this is one method of evaluating a company. Attention to detail behind their claims may reflect attention to detail throughout the company.

In 2004, the FDA approved a Qualified Health Claim on Omega-3 Fatty Acids and Coronary Heart Disease for food and supplements.

FDA Qualified Health Claim

Supportive but not conclusive research shows that consumption of EPA and DHA omega-3 fatty acids may reduce the risk of coronary heart disease. One serving of [name] provides [#] gram of EPA and DHA omega-3 fatty acids.

Docket No. 2003Q-0401

Learn more about the company whose product you recommend

You can learn a lot about a company by making a short phone call. Company websites can be useful, but they are usually limited to marketing information. Take a few minutes to call the company. Company contact information is on every product label and available on the Internet. Identify yourself, explain you'd like to learn more about their products and ask questions. Here are some questions that may be helpful in learning more about the company and products they sell:

- Do they have trained technical staff available for professional consult? In general, sales people are trained to sell.
- Do they have independent testing done on the finished product? If so, where can you see the results?

- Can they provide evidence for the claims they are making? If so, ask them to fax or email the information to you and review it.
- Do they do research with their product? Is that research published in scientific journals? If so, get the references or ask them to send it to you.
- Do they hire or work with healthcare professionals with training from accredited institutions? Non-accredited credentials are easy and inexpensive to get and many people don't know the difference. Colleagues, don't be fooled! Verify the credentials of those promoting products and then inform your clients with pertinent information. Verification can be done through an Internet search on the program supplying the credential. Brand markets frequently hire healthcare professionals to write or speak on their behalf, but that is different from being involved with research and development.

Dietary supplement companies like to know who is using and recommending the products they sell. Healthcare professionals expecting evidence-based information helps raise the bar for everyone.

STORING FISH OIL: CAPSULES VS. LIQUID

Fish oil supplements should contain antioxidants that serve as natural preservatives. It is not necessary to keep fish oil capsules in the freezer. Keeping them chilled isn't a bad idea, but it's not necessary. Liquid fish oil, on the other hand, must be stored in the refrigerator and is best consumed within a month. Advise clients using liquids to purchase quantities that they will consume within a month and, for certain, no longer than two months. Fish oil products (capsules or liquid) should never be exposed to high temperatures or light (e.g., don't leave them in the car on a hot day).

FISH BURPS OR REPEAT

A small percentage of people taking fish oil supplements report fishy burps or *repeat*. These usually can be alleviated. If your client reports burping, look first at the digestive health of your client. Do they have ongoing trouble with digestion? Is so, address it. Advise that they take the supplement with food, preferably their largest meal of the day. If they forget the supplement with their meal, recommend that they take it with their next meal and not on an empty stomach. Taking the supplement at bedtime may avoid fish burps.

Some believe taking the capsule when it is frozen reduces repeat. In actuality, it is more common for people to report burping with inexpensive fish oil capsules. For this reason, enteric-coated capsules may alleviate the problem. Trying a different brand or a different form (e.g., liquid) may also make the difference. People seldom report fishy burps when they take cod liver oil in liquid form. Not everyone experiences fishy burps but it is a barrier worth addressing, even if uncomfortable for the client to discuss.

Ease of daily supplementation is important because individuals who regularly experience repeat are less likely to be compliant over time and they will not receive the intended benefit from the supplement. A product that is affordable and pleasant to take will lead to success for both the provider and the client.

INDEPENDENT OR 3RD-PARTY TESTING

Omega-3 products can be independently tested to verify that the amount of EPA and DHA stated on the label is in the product. For better-quality fish oil products, this is not a problem. Products can also be tested to verify that they meet quality manufacturing standards for purity (removal of toxins) and freshness (not oxidized/rancid).

In regard to omega-3, there is a quality standard (the voluntary GOED Monograph) for fish oils, but it does not apply to cod liver oils or krill oils. There is a US Pharmacopeia (USP) standard for fish oils as well. Two programs that perform independent testing for omega-3 fish oils and report results are the International Fish Oil Standards (www.ifos-program.com) and Consumer Labs (www.consumerlab.com); access to Consumer Labs requires membership.

PRESCRIPTION FISH OIL

Lovaza® from GlaxoSmithKline is FDA-approved, along with diet, to reduce very high triglycerides (>500 mg/dl) in adults. Lovaza is composed of concentrated EPA and DHA omega-3 from fish oil. Each 4-capsule dose provides close to 3.4 grams of EPA and DHA.

There are many variations of omega-3 fatty acids in different stages of research and development for use as drugs. Examples include AMR101® and Epanova™. Medical indications under investigation extend beyond cardiovascular health, to arthritis, vision, and asthma, among others.

BORAGE, EVENING PRIMROSE, AND BLACK CURRANT OILS

Borage oil, evening primrose oil (EPO) and black currant oils are plant-based oils with a long history of traditional use, primarily among women. These oils are used in dietary supplements as a source of GLA (gamma linolenic acid) and are often blended with fish oil. GLA is an omega-6 fatty acid (18:3n-6) that occurs in the metabolic path between linoleic acid (18:2n-6) and arachidonic acid (20:4n-6). In theory, GLA could be beneficial but there is very little positive research in humans.

FREQUENTLY ASKED QUESTIONS

Are fish oil supplements safe and do they work?

This is the first question that should be asked about all dietary supplements. Getting EPA and DHA omega-3 from purified fish/marine/algal oil sources that is sold by reputable companies is one of the safest supplements on the market. And yes, they work. What they do and how well they do it will be determined by the dose and form recommended and by the client's compliance.

How do I choose one brand over another?

This is not easy to answer. Better-quality products taste better, and in my working experience, there are fewer complaints of fish burps with better quality products.

In general, better-quality fish oils products cost more to produce. Getting more long-chain omega-3 per capsule costs more because it costs more to concentrate. Use of natural stabilizers cost more than synthetic ones. Price is not the only indicator, but it is *an* indicator. Getting more EPA and DHA per capsule is often a better value.

Companies who are members of GOED have agreed to meet the international standards for fish oil manufacturing. A list of members can be found on the GOED website (www.goedomega3.com). Recommend brands from reputable companies. Learn about the companies.

For a moment, consider the "cost" of consuming degraded marine oil supplements, perhaps from oil that was not carefully filtered, or oil that was exposed to higher temperatures or didn't have enough antioxidants added to protect the oil; is there potential harm? It's possible. We know innately when a food has degraded and marine oils are sourced from food. Common sense here is a good guide.

What about my clients who buy fish oil supplements at wholesale or value stores?

Commend them for taking positive steps toward their health, and then have an honest discussion on how they want to spend their health dollars.

While there are exceptions, in general, fish oil products can be divided into three categories: 1) *better* products, 2) those that meet *minimum* standards, and 3) those to *avoid*. See the section on quality above.

- *Better* products are available at natural food stores, from other healthcare professionals and pharmacies.
- *Minimum* standard products are available at big box, wholesale, and chain stores.
- *Avoid* products are available at deep-discount wholesalers. Avoid them.

It's best to buy from sellers who know the source of their products. Frankly speaking, to get omega-3s from sustainably caught fish without destroying them in the process takes expensive equipment and considerable skill and these cost money. The same wide range of quality exists on the Internet, and perhaps to even greater extremes. For example, some of the freshest cod liver oil available can only be purchased over the Internet and there are also fish oil products shipped from unidentified or misrepresented places that should be avoided.

Remind your clients that the benefits of EPA and DHA are proven, and your goal for them is to have them eat fatty fish twice a week (at pennies on the dollar) or to be compliant with an agreeable supplement (for less than a dollar a day). If they meet this goal, it can improve their health and reduce their risk of death. Convenience in shopping or saving a few pennies isn't worth losing that chance.

Does buying purified marine oil supplements matter?

Yes. Consume marine oil products that are purified to a quality standard. In this instance, align with the professionals. Be alert to companies for whom claiming to be "more natural" translates into being less purified and then avoid their products.

What do I do if a capsule smells bad?

If a capsule smells or tastes bad, it probably is bad and should not be consumed. "Bad" usually means oxidized; that is, the oil was exposed to oxygen or high temperatures for too long, or poorly purified. The effect of consuming oxidized fish oil has not been well studied in humans, but reason and logic suggests that we avoid it. We don't eat bad fish, and we should not consume bad fish oil. If the bottle of capsules is new, return it to the store where you bought it. If it has been around a good while, discard it.

What is concentrated fish oil?

Concentrated fish oil is fish oil that has been concentrated to provide more EPA and DHA than naturally occurs in fish. Regular fish oil is about 30% omega-3 (e.g., a 1000-mg capsule provides about 300 mg EPA and DHA). Concentrated fish oil products contain 40–80% EPA and

DHA. Concentrations of 50–60% are common, so, for example, a 1000-mg capsule concentrated to 60% would provide 600 mg EPA and DHA; that is double the amount of EPA and DHA in regular fish oil but not usually double the price. Concentrated fish oil products are often a better value, and compliance may be better. Note that some discount companies use the word "concentrated" as a marketing term when the oil is regular 30% omega-3. Here is more reason to give specific advice on the dose of EPA and DHA and to read labels.

What should I tell clients who find the capsules difficult to swallow?

Some manufacturers use smaller capsules although in order to obtain the same amount of oil and omega-3s, clients need to take several capsules. Fish oil also comes in chewable capsules, flavored liquids (keep refrigerated), and in a pudding-like emulsion in individual pouches or bottles (must be refrigerated). Also consider which EPA and DHA fortified foods that the client likes to eat and will buy on a regular basis. A key determining factor in this decision is the reason for supplementation and the dose you are aiming for them to consume.

Can I recommend fish oil supplements to my clients who are on medications?

Sometimes yes and sometimes no. Research has shown that omega-3 fish oil supplements are beneficial to take in conjunction with some statin medicines, for example. In research trials on depression, fish oil supplements are sometimes used along with antidepressant medication with good results. Specifics on this are beyond the scope of this handbook but worth learning more about.

My clients like to buy organic. Can they get organic fish oil?

No, organic fish oil is not available as there is no organic standard for fish. The international standards that exist for fish and seafood are related to environmental and sustainability issues. For example, the Marine Stewardship Council (msc.org) is a non-profit organization that has standards for sustainability. Advising your clients to look for the MSC ecolabel™ on foods (not supplements) will support global sustainability.

What about my clients who must limit iodine?

Iodine is one of the elements removed during purification by better manufacturers but it is difficult to guarantee the complete absence of iodine. In my working knowledge of two fish oil suppliers, their concentrated fish oil has contained 0.5-1 mcg of iodine per gram of fish oil and not more than 2 mcg/gram. Dietary Reference Intake for adults is 150 mcg iodine per day[5]. Be sure to contact the company and get confirmation. Note that removing iodine is not required of manufacturers, so lower-quality fish oils could contain higher levels.

What do I do with clients who think fish oil and omega-3 are different?

Take the opportunity to teach them about essential fatty acids and tell them that fish oil is a source of the most functional forms of omega-3s. Then guide them to make sound dietary choices. In the process, you may be able to improve their diet and save them some money.

My client buys omega-3 fortified gummy candies for the whole family and I'm not sure how to advise.

Sugar-based chewable supplements typically contain a small amount of nutrients. Look at the dose of omega-3 per serving and the number of servings consumed by each family member (see Table 3-3). Consider their diet and the reason for taking the supplement. Do they eat any fish? Is the dose sufficient? Is the amount of sugar problematic, considering health status and other dietary habits? How much fish is consumed by the family? Consider if a discussion on the perception of vitamins as nutrients versus candy for children is relevant. Discuss and recommend other options if appropriate.

Is it possible to consume too much fish oil?

Use an evidence-based approach when advising clients. Keep in mind that genetic factors and health history can influence how a client responds to supplementation. Eskimos and the Japanese have consumed fish rich in omega-3s daily for centuries with little to no ill-effect and they have low rates of heart disease, the leading cause of death in most developed nations. And practically speaking, there is likely a tissue level at which one receives no additional health benefit. Much of what we have learned about omega-3 intervention has come from populations whose tissue levels of omega-3s are relatively low and the ability to reliably test an individual's omega-3 levels is relatively new.

On another note, in North America, it is standard procedure to stop taking fish oil supplements two weeks prior to surgery. The FDA has established a GRAS (Generally Regarded as Safe) level at 3 grams of EPA and DHA per day[6]. EPA and DHA blood cell membranes levels of 8% or higher reduce risk for death by heart disease. See Chapter 1 for more information.

What are omega 3-6-9 products?

The best value for the pocket book (and the body) is usually to supplement with EPA and DHA omega-3 instead of the 3-6-9 products. Here's why. First, omega-9 (oleic acid) naturally occurs in olive oil; it is healthful but not an essential fatty acid. Second, while omega-6 is an essential fatty acid, it is already abundant in the food supply so supplementing with them does not usually provide added benefit. That said, the form of omega-6 in these combination products may be GLA (gamma linolenic acid), for which there exists more anecdotal testimony than published evidence. There is some data suggesting that when GLA is taken in a particular fatty acid balance, it can reduce inflammation but that is not the typical ratio in the 3-6-9 blend.

This blend is popular among consumers because they believe they are doing the best for themselves. It may appear to be a better deal but it may not be the best value.

Should my client get supplements with GLA for her child with ADD?

No, it is not necessary. According to published research, there does not appear to be additional benefit from including GLA (gamma linolenic acid, an omega-6) in the child's supplement. Some supplements for children include GLA; this is based on old study findings and in actuality, the amount in the supplement may be so low that it is inconsequential. There isn't good evidence to support paying more for a product that contains GLA.

Of interest, one study completed in children with ADD that used DHA only had neutral findings. At this time, your best approach is an omega-3 supplement providing more EPA than DHA per serving. Aim for at least 500 mg total per day and more for older children.

ENDNOTES

1   Kris-Etherton PM, Innis S. Position of the American Dietetic Association and Dietitians of Canada: Dietary fatty acids. *J Am Dietetic Assn* 2007;107:1599-1611.

2   Kris-Etherton PM, et al. for the American Heart Association Nutrition Committee. Omega-3 fatty acids and cardiovascular disease: New recommendations from the American Heart Association. *Arterioscler Thromb Vasc Biol* 2003;23:151-152.

3   Freeman MP, et al. Omega-3 fatty acids: Evidence base for treatment and future research in psychiatry. *J Clin Psychiatry* 2006;67(12):1954-1967.

4   Omega-3 absorption pilot trial, unpublished data. Portland, Oregon, 2010.

5   Dietary Reference Intakes. Institute of Medicine, National Academy of Sciences, Food and Nutrition Board, Bethesda, MD.

6   Department of Health and Human Services. Substances affirmed as generally recognized as safe: Menhaden oil. 21 CFR Part 184. Food and Drug Administration. Federal Register, 1997;62(108):30751-30757.

NOTES

NOTES

Resources

RECOMMENDED INTAKE TABLES

American Dietetic Association and Dietitians of Canada: Omega-3 Fatty Acid Recommendations

Target population	Recommendation
General adult population	Omega-3 long-chain PUFA (EPA + DHA): 500 mg per day
General adult population	2 servings per week of preferably fatty fish • Approximately 9 oz of cooked fish per week provides 500 mg per day EPA + DHA
General adult population	Omega-3 PUFA-ALA: 0.6%–1.2% of energy (based on 2000 kcal diet) • 0.6%: 1.3 g • 0.9%: 2.0 g • 1.2%: 2.7 g

Source: Kris-Etherton PM, Innis S. Position of the American Dietetic Association and Dietitians of Canada. *J Am Diet Assoc* 2007;107:1599-1611.
Abbreviations: PUFA= poly-unsaturated fatty acid, ALA= alpha-linolenic acid, EPA= eicosapentaenoic acid, DHA= docosahexaenoic acid

American Heart Association Omega-3 Fatty Acid Recommendations

Target population	Recommendation
General adult population [1]	Consume fish, particularly fatty fish (mackerel, lake trout, herring, sardines, albacore tuna, salmon) ≥ 2 times per week.
	Consume plant-derived omega-3 fatty acids (tofu, soybeans, walnuts, flaxseeds, canola oil containing ALA).
Adults with documented coronary heart disease [1]	1 g of EPA + DHA per day obtained from consumption of oily fish or omega-3 fatty acid supplements.
Adults with hypertriglyceridemia [1]	2–4 g EPA + DHA may lower triglyceride 20–40%
	Use of > 3 g per day should be done only under physician care.
Women with hypercholesterolemia and/or hypertriglyceridemia [2]	For primary and secondary prevention, consider consumption of omega-3 fatty acids in the form of fish or in capsules (e.g., EPA 1800 mg/d).

Source: [1]Kris-Etherton PM, et al. Omega-3 fatty acids and cardiovascular disease: New recommendations from the American Heart Association. *Arterioscler Thromb Vasc Biol*, 2003;23:151-152.

[2]Mosca L, et al. Effectiveness-based guidelines for the prevention of cardiovascular disease in women 2011 update: A guideline from the American Heart Association. *Circulation* 2011;123:1243-1262.

Abbreviations: ALA= alpha-linolenic acid, EPA= eicosapentaenoic acid, DHA= docosahexaenoic acid

American Psychiatric Association Omega-3 Fatty Acid Recommendations

Target population	Recommendation
General adult population	Consume fish ≥2 times per week.
Patients with mood, impulse-control, or psychotic disorders	Consume 1 g EPA + DHA per day.
Patients with mood disorders	Supplement of 1-9 g per day may be useful.
	Use of > 3 g per day should be monitored by a physician.

Source: Freeman MP, et al. Omega-3 fatty acids: Evidence basis for treatment and future research in psychiatry. *J Clin Psychiatry* 2006;67:1954-1967.

Abbreviations: EPA= eicosapentaenoic acid, DHA= docosahexaenoic acid

Global and Select Countries: Omega-3 Fatty Acid Recommendations for the General Adult Population

Country / Region	Organization	Recommendation
Global	International Society for the Study of Fats and Lipids[1]	• DHA + EPA: 0.65 g/2000 kcal/d • DHA: at least 0.22 g/2000 kcal/d • EPA: at least 0.22 g/2000 kcal/d
Global	NATO workshop on omega-3 and omega-6 fatty acids[2]	800 mg EPA/DHA per day
Europe	Expert Workshop of the European Academy of Nutritional Sciences[3]	People who do not eat fish should consider consuming marine omega-3 PUFA equivalent to the amount obtained from fatty fish, namely 200 mg EPA + DHA daily
Europe	European Food Safety Agency[4]	250 mg EPA + DHA per day
Australia	National Heart Foundation of Australia[5]	500 mg EPA/DHA per day, obtained through fish, fish oil supplements, or enriched food for prevention of heart disease
Belgium	Belgian Superior Health Council[6]	Two servings of fatty fish
France	AFFSA[7]	• General Nutrition: 250 mg DHA per day, 250 mg EPA per day, 500 mg EPA + DHA per day
Japan	Ministry of Health, Labor and Welfare[8]	> 1 g EPA + DHA per day

Country / Region	Organization	Recommendation
Scandinavia	Nordic Council of Ministers[9]	• EPA + DHA: 450 mg per day • Total omega-3 PUFAs: 1.0% of energy per day
United Kingdom	British Nutrition Foundation[10]	• One to two portions of oil-rich fish per week, which will provide around 2–3 g of the very long chain omega-3 fatty acids • Weekly intake of 1.5 g of EPA + DHA
United States	Institute of Medicine[11]	• Men: 1.6 g per day of ALA, approximately 10% of which is EPA + DHA • Women: 1.1 g per day of ALA, approximately 10% of which is EPA + DHA

[1] Simopoulos AP, et al. Workshop statement of the essentiality of and recommended dietary intakes for Omega-6 and Omega-3 fatty acids. *Prostaglandins Leukot Essent Fatty Acids* 2000;63:119-121.

[2] Simopoulous AP. Summary of the NATO advanced research workshop on dietary w3 and w6 fatty acids: Biological effects and nutritional essentiality. *J Nutr* 1989;119:521-528.

[3] de Eckere EA, et al. Health aspects of fish and n-3 polyunsaturated fatty acids from plant and marine origin. *Eur J Clin Nut*, 1998;52:749-753.

[4] EFSA Panel on Dietetic Products, Nutrition, and Allergies (NDA). Scientific opinion on dietary reference values for fats, including saturated fatty acids, polyunsaturated fatty acids, monounsaturated fatty acids, trans fatty acids, and cholesterol. *EFSA J* 2010;8:1461. Available online: www.efsa.europa.eu

[5] National Heart Foundation of Australia. Position statement on fish, fish oils, n-3 polyunsaturated fatty acids and cardiovascular health. Presented at AIFST conference July 2008.

[6] Superior Health Council of Belgium. Recommendations and claims made on omega-3-fatty acids (SHC 7945). 2005.

[7]AFFSA (France). Avis de l'Agence française de sécurité sanitaire des aliments relatif à l'actualisation des apports nutritionnels conseillés pour les acides gras. Retrieved from: http://www.afssa.fr/cgi-bin/countdocs.cgi?Documents/NUT2006sa0359EN.pdf.

[8]Ministry of Health and Welfare, Japan. Recommended dietary allowances for Japanese, 6th ed. Tokyo: Daiichi-Shuppan, 1999.

[9]NNR (Nordic Nutrition Recommendations). 2004. Integrating nutrition and physical activity. Nord 2004:13. Nordic Council of Ministers, Copenhagen.

[10]British Nutrition Foundation Conference held on 1 December 1999 to draw attention to the briefing paper on "*n*-3 Fatty acids and Health."

[11]Institue of Medicine. Dietary reference intakes for energy, carbohydrate, fiber, fat, fatty acids, cholesterol, protein, and amino acids. National Academy of Sciences: Washington, DC, 2002.

Recommendations and Daily Intakes for DHA for Pregnant and Lactating Women

Daily intake recommendations

World Association of Perinatal Medicine recommends a minimum intake of 200 mg DHA/day[1,2]

Other expert recommendations: 300 – 900 mg DHA/day[3,4]

Note: More than 1000 mg DHA have been used in clinical research without adverse effects.

Current daily intake from published research

Average 70-80 mg DHA/day[5,6]

Average intake per food frequency questionnaire of both EPA & DHA among low-income pregnant women[7]:

- Overall: 39 mg/d
- African Americans: 93 mg/d
- Hispanics: 55 mg/d
- Caucasians: 31 mg/d

[1]Koletzko B, et al. The roles of long-chain polyunsaturated fatty acids in pregnancy, lactation and infancy: Review of current knowledge and consensus recommendations. *J Perinat Med* 2008;36:5-14.

[2]Koletzko B, et al. for the Perinatal Lipid Intake Working Group. Dietary fat intakes for pregnant and lactating women. *Br J Nutr* 2007;98:873-877.

[3]Simopoulos AP, et al. Workshop statement on the essentiality of and recommended dietary intakes for omega-6 and omega-3 fatty acids. *Prostaglandins Leukot Essent Fatty Acids* 2000;63:119-121.

[4]Hibbeln JR, Davis JM. Considerations regarding neuropsychiatric nutritional requirements for intakes of omega-3 high unsaturated fatty acids. *Prostaglandins Leukot Essent Fatty Acids* 2009;81:179-186.

[5]Denoome J, et al. Directly quantitated dietary (n-3) fatty acid intakes of pregnant Canadian women are lower than current dietary recommendations. *J Nutr* 2005;135:206-211.

[6]Stark KD, et al. Comparison of bloodstream fatty acid composition from African-American Women at gestation, delivery, and postpartum. *J Lipid Res* 2005;46:516-525.

[7]Nochera CL, et al. Consumption of DHA + EPA by low-income women during pregnancy and lactation. *Nutr Clin Pract* 2011;26:445-450.

*Recommendations and Daily Intakes for EPA and DHA for Children**

Daily intake recommendations**
1-2 fatty fish meals per week[1]
OR
Approximately 500 mg EPA and DAH per day[1]

Current daily intake from published research

	EPA	*DHA*	*Combined*
Children ages 4-8[2]	38 ± 9 mg	54 ± 11 mg	93 mg/d
Children ages 4-7[3]		37±63 mg	

* In lieu of formal recommendations for dietary intakes of EPA + DHA for children, experts recommend that dietary advice for children be consistent with advice for adults in order to reduce the risk for cardiovascular disease[1].

** The American Academy of Pediatrics[4] recommends that children "eat more fish, especially oily fish, broiled or baked introduced and regularly served as an entrée."

[1] Uauy R, Dangur AD. Fat and fatty acid requirements and recommendations for infants of 1-2 years and children of 2-18 years. *Ann Nutr Metab* 2009;55:76-96.

[2] Madden SMM, et al. Direct diet quantification indicates low intakes of (n-3) fatty acids in children 4 to 8 years old. *J Nutr* 2009;139:1-5.

[3] Lien VW, Clandinin MT. Dietary assessment of arachidonic acid and docosahexaenoic acid intake in 4-7 year-old children. *J Am Coll Nutr* 2009;28:7-15.

[4] Gidding SS, et al. Dietary recommendations for children and adolescents: A guide for practitioners. *Pediatrics* 2006;117:544-559.

GOED MANUFACTURING STANDARDS FOR FISH OIL*

Definition and scope

Supplements containing omega-3 fatty acids may contain predominantly DHA, EPA, or a combination. Supplements containing DHA or EPA as a single source report the content of omega-3 on a weight/weight basis or as mg of EPA or DHA per gram. When a mixture of the two is present, the amount of each may be reported separately or as a total mg of EPA and DHA per gram. Omega-3 products containing EPA and DHA are liquid at room temperature and range in color from pale yellow, light yellow, to orange. Manufacturing standards are applicable to EPA and DHA dietary supplements found in bulk oil and encapsulated oil products derived from fish, plant, or microbial sources (excluding cod liver oil) for the stated shelf-life of the product.

Identification

The first step is to identify that EPA and DHA are present in the supplement. Gas chromatography is a common type of assay used to separate and analyze compounds present in a mixture. From the assay, the presence of EPA and DHA are determined. The identity of the product is determined based on retention time comparison to established reference standards.

Freshness/Quality

To ensure the high quality of supplements, standard measures for freshness have been determined. The peroxide and anisidine values indicate freshness and represent oxidation of the product. TOTOX is a formula of peroxide and anisidine values and represents a combined maximum level for those levels as well as total oxidation of the product. Lower numbers are more desirable and indicate better freshness.

Maximum levels for these values:

- Peroxide value (PV): maximum 5 meq/kg; AOCS Official Method Cd8-53
- Anisidine value (AV): maximum 20; AOCS Official Method Cd-18-90
- TOTOX: Maximum 26 (result of calculation, [2xPV] + AV)

Purity

Standards have also been set for potential contaminants so that when buying omega-3 supplements, one can expect them to free of contaminants to a specified level. Environmental contaminants measured are dioxins (polychlorinated dibenzo-*para*-dioxins [PCDDs] and polychlorinated dibenzofurans [PCDFs]) and polychlorinated biphenyls [PCBs]. Standards for heavy metals, lead, cadmium, mercury, and arsenic, have also been established.

Standards* for potential contaminants are:

- PCDDs and PCDFs: Maximum 2 pg WHO-PCDD/F-TEQ/g
  ‣ Dioxin limits include the sum of PCDDs and PCDFs and are expressed in World Health Organization (WHO) toxic equivalents using WHO-toxic equivalent factors (TEQ). This means that analytical results relating to 17 individual dioxin congeners of toxicological concern

* *Adapted from the GOED Voluntary Monograph http://www.goedomega3.com/quality-standards.html

are expressed in a single quantifiable unit: TCDD toxic equivalent concentration or TEQ.

- PCBs: Maximum 0.09 mg/kg
  ‣ Total PCBs should be expressed on a weight/weight basis and should include IUPAC congeners 28, 52, 101, 118, 138, 153, and 180.
- Dioxin-like PCBs: Maximum 3 pg WHO-TEQ/g (maximum for dioxin and furans remains at 2 pg/g)
- Lead (Pb): less than 0.1 mg/kg
- Cadmium (Cd): less than 0.1 mg/kg
- Mercury (Hg): less than 0.1 mg/kg
- In-organic Arsenic (As): less than 0.1 mg/kg

WHERE THE STORY BEGINS: REFERENCES

Bang HO, Dyerberg J, Nielsen AB. Plasma lipid and lipo-protein pattern in Greenlandic west-coast Eskimos. *Lancet.* 1971;7701:1143-1146.

Bang HO, Dyerberg J, Hjorne N. The composition of food consumed by Greenland Eskimos. *Acta Med Scand.* 1976;200(1-2):69-73.

Dyerberg J, Bang HO, Hjorne N. Fatty acid composition of the plasma lipids in Greenland Eskimos. *Am J Clin Nutr.,* 1975;28(9):958-966.

ADDITIONAL RESOURCES
Environmental and sustainability
Marine Stewardship Council
www.msc.org

Monterey Bay Aquarium
http://www.montereybayaquarium.org/

EDF: Environmental Defense Fund
http://www.edf.org/
http://www.edf.org/oceans

Omega-3 blood testing
Holman Omega-3 Test®
http://www.omega3test.com

HS-Omega-3 Index®
http://www.omegaquant.com

Independent finished product testing
IFOS: International Fish Oil Standards
Testing Services: IFOS and QC Program
http://www.ifosprogram.com/ifos/testingservices.aspx

ConsumerLabs
Independent tests and reviews of vitamin, mineral, and
herbal supplements
http://www.consumerlab.com/

Manufacturing and quality standards
GOED Omega-3
Global organization for omega-3 EPA and DHA
www.geodomega3.com

Research

Office of Dietary Supplements: National Institutes of Health
http://ods.od.nih.gov/

PubMed: MEDLINE
Published research
PubMed: National Center for Biotechnological Information
http://www.ncbi.nlm.nih.gov/pubmed

International Omega-3 Learning and Education Consortium for Health and Medicine
www.omega3learning.uconn.edu

American Dietetics Association Evidence Analysis Library
http://www.adaevidencelibrary.com/default.cfm?auth=1

Plant-source omega-3s

Flax Council of Canada
http://www.flaxcouncil.ca/

Canola Council of Canada
http://www.canolacouncil.org/

Kelley Fitzpatrick, MS
NutriTech Consulting
kelleyf@shaw.ca

Useful Client Tools

These and other tools are available online.
Contact the author for more information
or visit www.omega3handbook.com.

Associations between Omega-3 Levels and Health

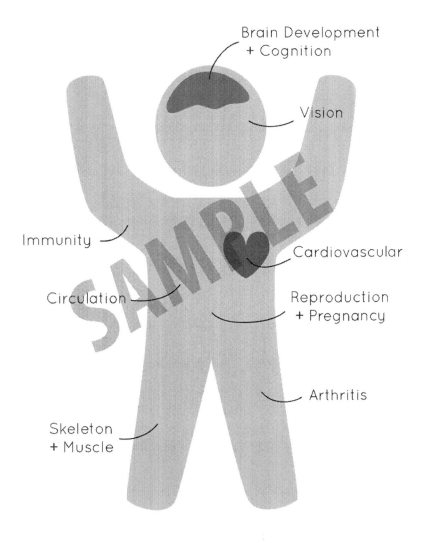

Brain Development + Cognition

Vision

Immunity

Cardiovascular

Circulation

Reproduction + Pregnancy

Arthritis

Skeleton + Muscle

Provider:

OMEGA-3 RECOMMENDATION

Name: _____

Date: _____

DOSE _____ g/d

FORM _____ EPA+DHA

DURATION _____

FOR _____

_____
Signature

How much do I need to eat daily
to get 500 mg EPA+DHA omega-3?

Each amount contains approximately 500 mg EPA + DHA omega-3*

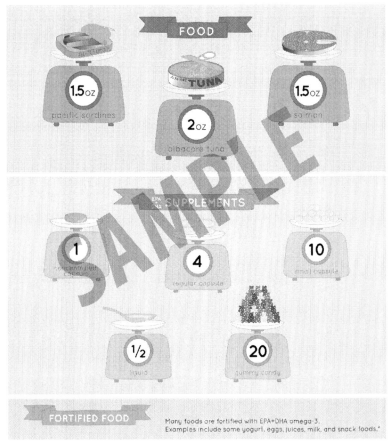

*Be sure to read the label.

Author's Bio and Contact Information

Gretchen Vannice, MS, RD, is an independent nutrition educator, trainer, and research specialist based in Portland, Oregon. She is an author and peer-reviewer for the Journal of the Academy of Nutrition and Dietetics. She has served as the chair of the International Science Committee, Global Organization for Omega-3 EPA and DHA (GOED) since 2007. A consultant to dietitians, health professionals, and the omega-3 industry, she is a frequent national speaker. You can contact Gretchen at gretchen@omega3handbook. com or 503-281-4287 or www.omega3rd.com

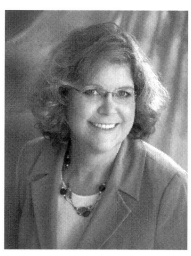

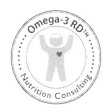

Photograph: Mark Comella

NOTES

NOTES

NOTES

NOTES

NOTES

NOTES

NOTES

13701114R00076

Made in the USA
Lexington, KY
15 February 2012